Ferroudja Djeghali
Nacima Kaci
Nassima Makhloufi

Perinatal asphyxia in term newborns

Ferroudja Djeghali
Nacima Kaci
Nassima Makhloufi

Perinatal asphyxia in term newborns

Diagnosis and management

ScienciaScripts

Cover image: www.ingimage.com

This book is a translation from the original published under ISBN 978-620-6-71934-2.

Publisher:
Sciencia Scripts
is a trademark of
Dodo Books Indian Ocean Ltd. and OmniScriptum S.R.L publishing group

120 High Road, East Finchley, London, N2 9ED, United Kingdom
Str. Armeneasca 28/1, office 1, Chisinau MD-2012, Republic of Moldova, Europe
Printed at: see last page
ISBN: 978-620-7-95177-2

Foreword

The arrival of a child is an extraordinary event, a celebration of life and hope. Yet this miracle can sometimes be overshadowed by unforeseen complications, one of the most dreaded being perinatal asphyxia. This term, often synonymous with drama and uncertainty, refers to a lack of oxygen to the newborn during pregnancy or childbirth, with potentially serious and irreversible consequences.

Fortunately, advances in medicine and research are enabling us to better understand and apprehend this complex phenomenon. This book, the fruit of rigorous research, is an indispensable guide for anyone wishing to explore the ins and outs of perinatal asphyxia.

Whether you're a healthcare professional, a concerned parent or simply want to broaden your knowledge, these pages will shed valuable light on the various facets of this problem. You'll discover the causes and mechanisms of perinatal asphyxia, as well as the various diagnostic approaches for identifying and assessing its impact on the newborn.

As well as providing information and raising awareness, this book is also a message of hope. It highlights the considerable progress made in the prevention, diagnosis and management of perinatal asphyxia, offering a positive outlook for parents and healthcare professionals alike.

In conclusion, this book is an invaluable resource for all those wishing to learn about, understand and take action in the face of perinatal asphyxia. Its wealth of information, clear explanations and human approach make it a real reference tool, helping to lift the veil on this medical challenge and offer a better future to the most fragile newborns.

Dive into the following pages and let the light of knowledge shine on you.

Together, we can unlock the mysteries of perinatal asphyxia and give today's and tomorrow's children the chance of a healthy future.

Summary

This comprehensive book offers an in-depth overview of perinatal asphyxia, covering the following aspects:

- **Definition and pathophysiology :**

  A clear explanation of perinatal asphyxia, defined as impaired placental fetal gas exchange during childbirth; the underlying physiological processes that result.

- **Causes and risk factors :**

  A detailed discussion of the various factors that can increase the risk of perinatal asphyxia, such as maternal complications, placental problems and difficulties during delivery.

- **Clinical manifestations and diagnosis** :

  Presentation of clinical signs and diagnostic methods used to identify perinatal asphyxia, including Apgar score, blood gas analysis, electroencephalography and brain imaging.

- **Management and resuscitation :**

  A comprehensive guide to the management and resuscitation measures used to treat newborns suffering from perinatal asphyxia, such as assisted ventilation and therapeutic hypothermia.

- **Complications and prognosis :**

  A discussion of the potential complications associated with perinatal asphyxia, such as brain damage, multivisceral complications, as well as the long-term prognosis for affected neonates.

Collaborators :

- Benbouabdellah Malika Professor of Pediatrics
- Batouche Djamila Djahida, Head of Neonatal Pediatric Intensive Care Unit

Table of contents

Introduction

Perinatal asphyxia (PSA) is a public health problem, and a serious complication of childbirth. It is, in fact, a cause of high mortality and morbidity in newborns.

Worldwide, 2.5 million newborns die every year, accounting for 47% of all deaths among children under 5. Three quarters of neonatal deaths occur within the first week of life, and the highest risk of death is within the first 24 hours (1,2).

Perinatal asphyxia is responsible for 23% of deaths in the neonatal period, resulting in the death of around one million newborns worldwide every year (1,3).

The World Health Organization (WHO) defines neonatal asphyxia as the failure to establish or initiate normal breathing at birth (4). It is associated with marked impairment of uteroplacental gas exchange before or at the time of delivery, and if prolonged, leads to progressive hypoxemia, hypercapnia and significant metabolic acidosis (5). This may be prolonged partial asphyxia, sudden subtotal asphyxia due to a sentinel event, or a combination of both (6).

The combination of hypoxia and ischemia leads to a cascade of biochemical changes in the body, resulting in neuronal death and brain damage, with short-term consequences (hypoxo-anoxic encephalopathy, multivisceral failure) that can be life-threatening, but also long-term consequences, the most dreaded of which is cerebral palsy (CP), as well as mental retardation and epilepsy, with detrimental long-term consequences for the child and his or her family (7) .

In developed countries, improved primary obstetric care, effective neonatal resuscitation and therapeutic hypothermia have considerably improved the prognosis of this condition. In recent years, there has been a considerable reduction in the neonatal mortality rate, and in the incidence of APN. The latter does not exceed 2/1000 live births (NV) (8). The consequences of this pathology are even more serious in developing countries, where access to quality maternal and neonatal care is limited. The incidence rate is up to 10 times higher (9).

APN can be caused by antepartum events such as pre-eclampsia, primiparity, hypothyroidism, diabetes, extreme maternal age and infertility treatment (10-11); or intrapartum events including induction of labor, premature rupture of membranes >12h, acute labor injury, emergency cesarean section, instrumental extraction (12,13-16). Other studies report fetal-related factors such as low birth weight, gestational age, sex and fetal presentation (17-19).

To date, in the absence of effective pharmacological treatment, only therapeutic hypothermia (TH) has demonstrated efficacy in children with anoxemic encephalopathy, despite steady progress in the field of research (20,21).

The outcome of asphyxia depends above all on the quality of care provided. The care given to the newborn shortly after birth will also have a major influence on reducing the serious consequences of hypoxia.

Early assessment of the severity of an acute brain injury induced by hypoxoischemic encephalopathy (HIE) can be very useful for the prevention or treatment of these newborns.

Chapter 1

1. Definitions

1 .1. Acute fetal distress

Acute fetal distress (AFD) is a term commonly used in medical practice, which should no longer be the case as it has no precise definition. It traditionally refers to acute fetal hypoxia occurring during labor due to insufficient fetal-maternal gas exchange, suspected in the presence of an abnormal fetal heart rate (FHR). These abnormalities are found in almost a third of deliveries, whereas cord blood acidosis is much rarer (22); they are often the expression of adaptation to physiological states or reactions to aggression, trauma or drug exposure. For this reason, the term non-reassuring fetal state is preferred to acute fetal distress, in order to reduce the rate of unnecessary caesarean sections (23).

1.2. Fetal acidosis

Fetal acidosis is the biological parameter reflecting acute fetal hypoxia during labor. It is defined by an umbilical artery pH below 7.00 at birth. If it is associated with a base deficit (BD) in excess of 12 mmol/l, we speak of metabolic acidosis. It complicates around five out of every 1,000 deliveries (23). In 1994, the American College of Obstetricians and Gynecologists (ACOG) endorsed a pH threshold of 7.00, which has since been adopted by most clinical practice guidelines in other countries (24).

1.3. Fetal asphyxia per partum

The term asphyxia is experimentally defined as an alteration in respiratory gas exchange accompanied by the development of metabolic acidosis. It is generally reserved for experimental situations in which these changes can be established with precision. In the clinical context, fetal asphyxia is progressive hypoxemia and hypercapnia accompanied by significant metabolic acidemia (25). It is defined as fetal metabolic acidosis, which can be detected in cord blood. It is reflected in poor adaptation to extra-uterine life (disturbance of the Apgar score), signs of neonatal encephalopathy and/or signs of multivisceral failure in the first few days of life (23,26). In practice, all the diagnostic criteria for APN are rarely met: moderately altered early gasometry not available, Apgar score not collapsed, or uncertain anamnesis. In these situations, and especially if the acute obstetrical event is lacking, it is important to rule out other possible causes of this encephalopathy: traumatic, metabolic, genetic, infectious pathologies (27).

1.4. Neonatal encephalopathy

It is defined by the American Academy of Pediatrics (AAP) as the set of clinical manifestations reflecting the disruption of neurological function in the first days of life in a newborn at 35 weeks gestational age or more. It is manifested in varying degrees by disorders of tone and consciousness, as well as hyperexcitability, abnormal movements and convulsions (5).

1.5. Anoxic-ischemic encephalopathy (AIE)

It is the clinical translation of central nervous system damage secondary to perinatal asphyxia (28).

The clinical picture of EAI is not specific. Diagnosis is based on a number of clinical, biological and radiological parameters. Only 50% of encephalopathies are due to APN.

Among cerebral palsies in full-term infants, 20% are attributable to perinatal asphyxia (28). Scientific criteria are therefore needed to establish a causal link between perinatal asphyxia and cerebral palsy. This has been the subject of a multidisciplinary consensus based on an exhaustive review of the literature, defining the criteria for attributing neonatal encephalopathy or cerebral palsy to per partum asphyxia:

The American College of Obstetricians and Gynecologists (ACOG) and the American Academy of Pediatrics (AAP) issued the first statement in 1993, which included the following criteria (30):

- Profound metabolic acidosis (pH<7)
- Apgar score ≤3 at 5 min
- Neonatal encephalopathy
- Dysfunction of several organ systems

The second statement was approved by the International Cerebral Palsy Task Force in 1999 (25), revisited by AAP,and ACOG in 2003 (28) and in 2014 and reaffirmed in 2019 (5).The diagnostic criteria combine criteria
and inseparable clinical criteria:

Essential criteria

1. Evidence of fetal metabolic acidosis perpartum, at the cord over the umbilical artery or early in the newborn (less than one hour of life): pH < 7.00 and base deficit ≥ 12 mmol/l
2. Moderate to severe early encephalopathy in newborns of 34 weeks' gestation or more
3. Spastic quadriplegia or dyskinetic cerebral palsy

4. Exclusion of other causes: trauma, coagulation disorders, infectious pathology, genetic problem

- **Criteria that together suggest a perpartum origin but are not specific in themselves:**

(If some of the following criteria are absent or contradictory, the perpartum origin of the process remains uncertain)

1. Sentinel hypoxic event occurring before or during labor

(Abrupt and prolonged alteration of the fetal heart rate following the sentinel event, the trace preceding the event being normal; the evocative fetal heart rate abnormalities being bradycardia or disappearance of variability or late or prolonged variable decelerations)

2. Apgar score between 0 and 3 beyond five minutes.
3. Early multi-organ alterations (onset before 72 hours of age)
4. Early neonatal imaging showing non-focal anomalies

Reference

1. Wang H, Liddell CA, Coates MM, Mooney MD, Levitz CE, Schumacher AE, et al. Global, regional, and national levels of neonatal, infant, and under-5 mortality during 1990-2013: a systematic analysis for the Global Burden of Disease Study 2013. The Lancet. Sept 2014;384(9947):957-79.

2. UN-IGME-child-mortality-report-2019.pdf https://www.unicef.org/media/60561/file/UN-IGME-child-mortality-report-2019.pdf

3. Lawn JE, Blencowe H, Oza S, You D, Lee AC, Waiswa P, et al. Every Newborn: progress, priorities, and potential beyond survival. The Lancet]. july 2014 ;384(9938):189-205.

4. World Health Organizations .WHO_RHT_MSM_98.1.pdf https://apps.who.int/iris/bitstream/handle/10665/63953/WHO_RHT_MSM_98.1.pdf

5. Executive summary: Neonatal encephalopathy and neurologic outcome, second

edition. Report of the American College of Obstetricians and Gynecologists' Task Force on Neonatal Encephalopathy. Obstet Gynecol. 2014 Apr;123(4):896-901.

6. Ahearne CE, Boylan GB, Murray DM. Short and long term prognosis in perinatal asphyxia: An update. World J Clin Pediatr [Internet]. 8 Feb 2016 ;5(1):67-74.

7. Azra Haider B, Bhutta ZA. Birth asphyxia in developing countries: current status and public health implications. Curr Probl Pediatr Adolesc Health Care. 2006 ;36(5):178-88.

8. Kurinczuk JJ, White-Koning M, Badawi N. Epidemiology of neonatal encephalopathy and hypoxic-ischaemic encephalopathy. Early Hum Dev. June 2010 ;86(6):329-38.

9. Desalew A, Semahgn A, Tesfaye G. Determinants of birth asphyxia among newborns in Ethiopia: A systematic review and meta-analysis. Int J Health Sci. 2020 ;14(1).

10. Martinez-Biarge M, Diez-Sebastian J, Wusthoff CJ, Mercuri E, Cowan FM. Antepartum and Intrapartum Factors Preceding Neonatal Hypoxic-Ischemic Encephalopathy. PEDIATRICS. 1 Oct 2013 ;132(4):e952-9.

11. Azam M, Malik F, Khan P. Birth asphyxia risk factors. The professional. 2004;11(4):416-23.

12. Liljestrom L, Wikstrom AK, Agren J, Jonsson M. Antepartum risk factors for moderate to severe neonatal hypoxic ischemic encephalopathy: a Swedish national cohort study. Acta Obstet Gynecol Scand. May 2018;97(5):615-23.

13. Souza ALS de, Souza NL de, França DF de, Oliveira SIM de, Araújo AKC, Dantas DNA. Risk Factors for Perinatal Asphyxia in Newborns Delivered at Term. Open J Nurs. 8 Jul 2016 ;6(7):558-64.

14. Aslam HM, Saleem S, Afzal R, Iqbal U, Saleem SM, Shaikh MWA, et al. "Risk factors of birth asphyxia". Ital J Pediatr. Dec 2014;40(1):94.

15. Badawi N, Kurinczuk JJ, Keogh JM, Alessandri LM, O'Sullivan F, Burton PR, et al. Intrapartum risk factors for newborn encephalopathy: the Western Australian casecontrol study. BMJ. Dec 5 1998;317(7172):1554-8.

16. Yohannes Kibret, Getachew Hailu, Kassawmar Angaw. Determinants of BirthAsphyxia among Newborns in Dessie Town Hospitals, North-Central Ethiopia, 2018 International Journal of Sexual Health and Reproductive Health Care Open Access. 2019 Feb 2022; .2.2.22818.48328

17. Lee AC, Mullany LC, Tielsch JM, Katz J, Khatry SK, LeClerq SC, et al. Risk factors for neonatal mortality due to birth asphyxia in southern Nepal: a prospective, community-based cohort study. Pediatrics. 2008 ;121(5):e1381-90.

18. Torres AR, Naranjo JD, Salvador C, Mora M, Papazian O. [Predominant factors of neonatal encephalopathy: hypoxic and ischemia, a global problem]. Medicina (Mex). 2019;79 Suppl 3:15-9.

19. Mehar MF, Khan MA, Saleem R, Zafar F, Naqqash AB, Shahid S, et al. Risk factors of perinatal asphyxia at Nishtar Hospital Multan. Prof Med J. March 10,

2020;27(03):487-92.

20. Zhou W hao, Cheng G qiang, Shao X mei, Liu X zhi, Shan R bing, Zhuang D yi, et al. Selective head cooling with mild systemic hypothermia after neonatal hypoxic-ischemic encephalopathy: a multicenter randomized controlled trial in China. J Pediatr. sept 2010;157(3):367-72, 372.e1-3.

21. Gluckman PD, Wyatt JS, Azzopardi D, Ballard R, Edwards AD, Ferriero DM, et al. Selective head cooling with mild systemic hypothermia after neonatal encephalopathy: multicentre randomised trial. The Lancet 19 Feb 2005;365(9460):663-70

22. Low JA. Intrapartum fetal asphyxia: Definition, diagnosis, and classification. Am J Obstet Gynecol. May 1997;176(5):957-9.

23. Levy G, Bednarek N, Gabriel R. Per partum fetal asphyxia and nonassuring fetal states. 1 Jul 2014 ;5-077-A-30.

24. ACOG practice bulletin. Antepartum fetal surveillance. Number 9, October 1999 (replaces Technical Bulletin Number 188, January 1994). Clinical management guidelines for obstetrician-gynecologists. Int J Gynaecol Obstet Off Organ Int Fed Gynaecol Obstet. Feb 2000;68(2):175-85.

25. MacLennan A. A template for defining a causal relation between acute intrapartum events and cerebral palsy: international consensus statement. BMJ. 16 Oct 1999;319(7216):1054-9.

26. Zupan Simunek V. Definition of intrapartum asphyxia and consequences on outcome. Rev Sage-Femme . mai 2008 ;7(2):79-86.

27. Zupan Simunek V. Perinatal asphyxia at term: diagnosis, prognosis, elements of neuroprotection. Arch Pediatrics. May 2010;17(5):578-82.

28. Saliba E, Norbert K, Cantagrel S. Neuroprotection by hypothermia of hypoxic-ischemic encephalopathy in the term newborn. Réanimation [Internet]. 1 Nov 2010 ;19(7):655-64.

29. Hankins G. Defining the pathogenesis and pathophysiology of neonatal encephalopathy and cerebral palsy. Obstet Gynecol [Internet]. Sept 2003;102(3):628-36.

30. Carter BS, Haverkamp AD, Merenstein GB. The Definition of Acute Perinatal Asphyxia. Clin Perinatol. June 1, 1993 ;20(2):287-304.

Chapter 2

1. Physiology of maternal-fetal gas exchange during pregnancy

1.1. Oxygen (O_2) and the placental interventricular chamber

Normal fetal oxygenation is conditioned by maternal factors (maternal respiration, circulation and hematosis), fetal factors (fetal circulation and metabolism) and placental factors (placental vascularization and exchange).

Gas exchange in the inter-ventricular chamber (placental barrier) bears some resemblance to that observed at the pulmonary level.

Fetal blood is transported to the placenta via the umbilical artery. Umbilical arterial blood is characterized by a low concentration of oxygen and a high concentration of carbon dioxide. Oxygen from maternal blood crosses the placenta by a simple or facilitated diffusion process. It diffuses easily from the maternal circulation into the fetal circulation to bind to high-affinity fetal hemoglobin. Oxygen is captured, while carbon dioxide is eliminated from fetal blood by diffusion through the fine capillaries of the fetal placenta. This enables the fetus to withstand non-pathological hypoxia[i] [(1)].

1.2. Metabolism and fetal growth

The fetal brain needs a constant supply of energy in the form of ATP, which is obtained by metabolizing lactate, ketone bodies and glucose.

Under normal conditions, fetal energy metabolism is essentially aerobic, despite a physiologically low pO2 at the level of the umbilical vein (20-30 mmHg). Energy production is then particularly efficient, with a yield of 36 ATP molecules from one molecule of maternal glucose, but amino acids are also primarily oxidized to supply energy to the placenta and the fetus, enabling good fetal growth (1,2).

1.3. Mechanism of fetal adaptation to hypoxia

Reduced maternal-fetal gas exchange can occur during labor, leading to hypoxemia, hypoxia or even fetal asphyxia. Initially, this deterioration leads to hypoxemia (decrease in fetal arterial pO2).

The fetus initially adapts to this situation by improving placental oxygen extraction and decreasing its metabolic activity, preserving only its energy metabolism at the expense, in the longer term, of its growth in height and weight. When hypoxemia is prolonged, hypoxia (tissue oxygen depletion) eventually occurs. The fetus can still compensate for this situation by modifying the distribution of blood flow to its various organs.

The release of catecholamines causes peripheral vasoconstriction and redistribution of blood to the brain and heart, whose function is thus maintained as a priority. On the other hand, peripheral tissue metabolism becomes anaerobic, and lactic acid production leads to fetal metabolic acidosis.

When this acidosis is no longer compensated, the redistribution of blood flow to the brain and heart disappears. This leads to asphyxia and the possibility of neurological damage, poly visceral failure and death if the fetus is not extracted (1).

2. Pathophysiology of perinatal asphyxia

APN brain damage evolves over hours, days or even months. It follows a temporal sequence of brain lesions that can be divided into 3 phases **(figure 1).**

2.1. Primary energy failure

It occurs immediately after hypoxic-ischemic injury. Insufficient blood supply from the placenta causes hypoxic-ischemic damage to fetal tissue, impairing cardiac contractility. This leads to systemic hypotension and reduced cerebral blood flow.

The supply of oxygen and glucose to the brain is disrupted, triggering an alternative energy pathway known as anaerobic metabolism. This inefficient pathway leads to reduced energy production (ATP) and increased lactic acid accumulation. The result is a concomitant depolarization of the nerve membrane and an influx of calcium into the cells.

Thanks to calcium transporters, there is a pronounced release of excitatory amino acids (EAAs), such as glutamate, into the extracellular space. Buffering and cellular reabsorption of these EAAs requires energy, but due to energy depletion, high levels of EAAs accumulate, leading to glutamate neurotoxicity.

There is also a release of enzymes (peroxidases), which degrade the neuronal membrane. The combination of lactic acidosis, glutamate release, lipid peroxidation and the toxic effects of excitatory amino acids and nitrogenous substances leads to cell death known as necrosis (3-5).

2.2. Latent phase

Partial recovery follows 30 to 60 minutes after primary energy failure. It lasts 1 to 6 hours and is characterized by the recovery of mitochondrial oxidative metabolism, but with the continuation of inflammation and the apoptotic cascade.

Newborns with mild HIE will recover in this phase, but those with moderate or severe HIE will progress to the second phase. The latency phase is a window during which treatment options such as therapeutic hypothermia can be implemented to prevent progression of lesions to the second phase (5,6,7).

2.3. Secondary energy failure

A phase of secondary energy failure occurs 7 to 72 hours after the hypoxic-ischemic insult. Brain reperfusion occurs, accompanied by an explosion of excitatory transmitters and free radicals. Mitochondrial dysfunction worsens and ATP reserves are critically depleted. As the phase progresses, the mitochondria release cytochrome C and the cascade of lesions is reactivated and nerve cell apoptosis begins. Inflammatory factors such as cytokines are released, and brain damage becomes more extensive. Epileptic seizures are often apparent during this phase (6,7).

2.4. Energy failure in the commercial sector

Considered responsible for the permanent damage that persists into adulthood. It can last for months or even years after the hypoxic-ischemic event. Depending on the severity of the AIA and the response to the various therapeutic interventions, there are two possible outcomes. The first is recovery, where brain tissue enters a repair process and surviving nerves and glial cells begin to differentiate, proliferate and regenerate. However, if the injury is severe, damaged tissue continues to deteriorate as inflammation persists. Support cells, such as glia and astrocytes, continue to release harmful cytokines, leading to further neuronal death (6).

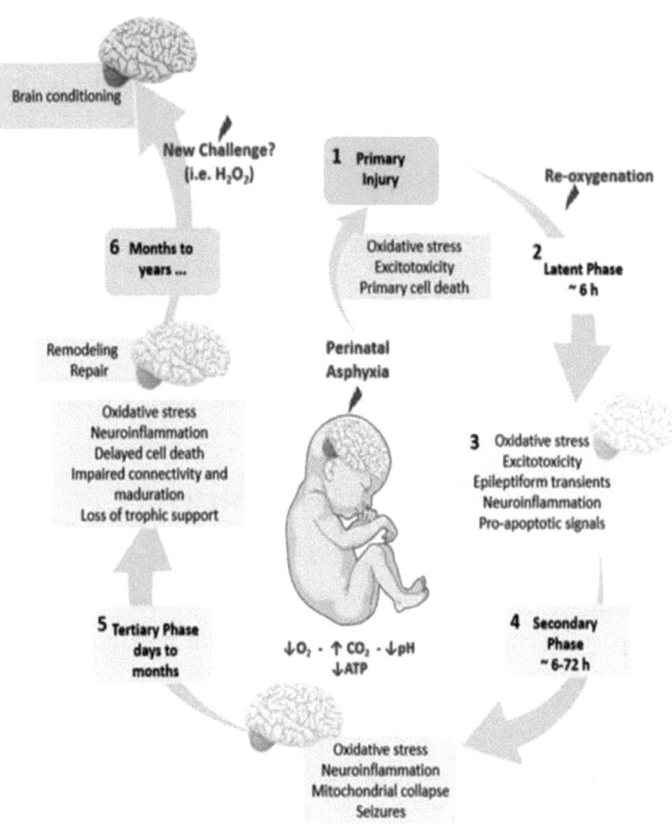

Figure 1: *The pathophysiological cascade caused by perinatal asphyxia (6)*

References :

1. Rainaldi MA, Perlman JM. Pathophysiology of Birth Asphyxia. Clin Perinatol 1 Sep 2016 ;43(3):409-22.

2. Mota-Rojas D, Villanueva-García D, Solimano A, Muns R, Ibarra-Ríos D, Mota-Reyes A. Pathophysiology of Perinatal Asphyxia in Humans and Animal Models. Biomedicines. 1 Feb 2022];10(2):347.

3. Greco P, Nencini G, Piva I, Scioscia M, Volta CA, Spadaro S, et al. Pathophysiology of hypoxic-ischemic encephalopathy: a review of the past and a view on the future. Acta Neurol Belg. Apr 2020;120(2):277-88.

4. Yildiz EP, Ekici B, Tatli B. Neonatal hypoxic ischemic encephalopathy: an update on disease pathogenesis and treatment. Expert Rev Neurother.

5. Ma. Esterlita Villanueva Uy, M.D.Neonatal-HIE-Pathophysiology-Features_WP.pdf

6. Moral Sánchez Y, Robertson NJ, Goñi de Cerio F, Alonso Alconada D. Neonatal hypoxia-ischemia: cellular and molecular bases of brain damage and therapeutic modulation of neurogenesis. Reverend Neurol. 2019 ;68(01):23.

7. MacLennan A. A template for defining a causal relation between acute intrapartum events and cerebral palsy: international consensus statement. BMJ. 16 Oct 1999;319(7216):1054-9.May 2017;17(5):449-59.

Chapter 3

1. Diagnosis of asphyxia

1.1. Diagnosis in utero

1.1.1. Fetal assessment on admission

Maternal and fetal condition must be assessed after admission to the onset of labor, by studying pregnancy follow-up records and looking for medical and obstetric history (IUGR, post-maturity, known oligo- or hydramnios, meconium fluid, premature rupture of membranes, etc.), which determines a higher level of fetal surveillance. The presence of abnormal signs on examination (decreased fetal movements, metrorrhagia, etc.), induce heightened vigilance in assessing fetal condition (1).

1.1.2. Pinard stethoscope auscultation

Intermittent monitoring of fetal heart rate using the Pinard stethoscope is a standard feature of obstetrical practice. It enables the heart to be auscultated, perceiving BCFs at frequencies ranging from 120 to 160 bpm. It requires precise counting and the reconstruction (in writing) of a true RCF curve. It requires the midwife's almost - permanent presence at the patient's bedside. Auscultation must be performed for 30 seconds, after a contraction and at a frequency of every 15 minutes during the first phase of labor, then every 5 minutes during the second phase. These conditions are not always met, which is why other means of monitoring fetal heart rate are so important (2).

1.1.3. The partogram

It is an inexpensive graphic representation of maternal and fetal observations recorded during the active phase of childbirth. It is a tool for continuous assessment of midwifery practice. Its use is recommended for labor monitoring, helping to identify labor anomalies and intervene appropriately to prevent prolonged labor (3). The use and performance of the partogram was significantly associated with a reduction in the incidence of birth asphyxia, according to the results of a retrospective study carried out in Ghana (4).

1.1.4. Meconium amniotic fluid

The appearance of the amniotic fluid is an essential element in clinical monitoring of labor. Meconium is normally emitted in the first twenty-four to forty-eight hours of life. The color of the amniotic fluid may change during labor. The fluid is said to be "stained" when it is yellowish or light-green with no particles, and "meconium" when it is brown-green, loaded with meconium particles. The passage of the contents of the fetal rectal ampulla into the amniotic fluid follows activation of the sympatho-adrenergic system, with fetal tachycardia. The presence of meconium fluid is not synonymous with asphyxia; it is a warning sign, but non-specific.
The results of different studies are divergent concerning the risk of fetal hypoxia occurring in the presence of meconium amniotic fluid. Indeed, compared with a control group with clear fluid, some show little or no difference in outcomes related to neonatal morbidity and mortality (pH at birth or Apgar score at 5ème minutes) (5,6). However, others conclude that non-reassuring fetal states are 3.5 times more frequent when the fluid is meconium, with a significant difference (7,8).
Souza A et al, in France (9), in a case-control study, concluded that the occurrence of severe neonatal metabolic acidosis was no more frequent in cases of evidence of stained or meconium-rich amniotic fluid. However, they did note an increase in the frequency of fetal heart rate abnormalities, which are responsible for an increase in the use of scalp pH, instrumental extractions and caesarean section.

1.1.5. Fetal heart rate analysis (ERCF)

The FHR has been used as a screening tool since the 1970s. It provides information on fetal well-being during pregnancy, labor and delivery. It reflects the balance between the sympathetic and parasympathetic systems. Its monitoring determines the state of fetal oxygenation. It can be used to detect abnormalities, but never to make a diagnosis (excellent negative predictive value, poor positive predictive value). In this case, 2nd-line methods are required (10).

Analysis of the FHR trace should be systematic, regular and noted on the par- togram. The quality of RCF recording and uterine contractions is essential for correct analysis of uterine activity anomalies, and for interpretation of the RCF, its analysis must be continuous from the active phase of labor (from 3 cm dilatation).

. Four basic criteria are used to analyze the RCF (1) :

➤ **Basic rhythm**

The basic rhythm is said to be normal between 110 and 160 beats per minute (bpm).

- Tachycardia is defined as a rhythm exceeding 160 bpm for more than 10 minutes.
- Bradycardia is defined as a rhythm below 110 bpm for more than 10 minutes.

➤ **Variability**

RCF variability is said to be absent when it is not visible (less than 2 bpm); minimal if less than or equal to 5 bpm; moderate or normal (between 6 and 25 bpm) and marked above 25 bpm.

➤ **Reactivity**

It is defined by the presence of accelerations. These correspond to a sudden rise in the FHR (≥15 bpm) with an abrupt slope. This episodic change lasts 15 seconds or more (but less than two minutes). Acceleration is said to be prolonged if it lasts between two and ten minutes.

➤ **Slowing down**

Slowdowns (or decelerations) are most often related to uterine contractions. Their amplitude is greater than 15 bpm and their duration greater than 15 seconds but less than two minutes. Decelerations are classified as early, variable, late and prolonged. The RCF is said to be normal when it meets the following four criteria:

- Basic rhythm: between 110 and 160 bpm
- Variability: between 6 and 25 bpm
- Reactivity: presence of accelerations
- Slowing down: absence

The classification of the National Institute of Child Health and Human Development (NICHD) (11), which is very simple, distinguishes three categories of layouts:

➤ **Category 1**: corresponds to tracings at low risk of acidosis, which include normal tracings, but also isolated early slowing, since the latter is not a sign of hypoxia.

➤ **Category 3:** corresponds to abnormal tracings with a high risk of acidosis, requiring immediate extraction.

➤ **Category 2**: includes all layouts that do not correspond to either category 1 or category 3: these are the so-called "intermediate" or "non-reassuring" layouts.

The NICHD considered the following combinations to be at high risk of fetal acidosis, requiring immediate fetal extraction:

- Repeated late decelerations and absent variability

- Repeated variable slowdowns and absent variability
- Persistent bradycardia and absent variability
- Persistent severe bradycardia.

The more complex CNGOF classification distinguishes four classes of FCR anomalies: "low-risk", "high-risk", "significant-risk" and "major-risk" for acidosis (12).

CNGOF anomalies "at major risk of acidosis" correspond to NICHD category 3:

- Persistent bradycardia and absent variability
- Sudden severe bradycardia (< 90 bpm)

-Repeated late, variable or prolonged slowdowns associated with absent variability

-Sequence of hon, successively comprising progressive tachycardia, minimal variability, loss of acceleration, then deceleration.

1.1.6. Second-line tests

1.1.6.1. Scalp pH

First proposed by Saling in 1961, it is indicated during labor in all situations of pathological FHR, accompanied by evidence of possible fetal hypoxia. The sampling technique requires rupture of the membranes, cervical dilatation of at least 2 or 3 cm and a cephalic fetal position. Fetal blood sampling is performed through a micro-incision in the scalp, using a specific needle or microblade (13).

Despite insufficient data demonstrating a benefit in newborns, scalp pH remains the second-line reference method, as it directly measures the criteria defining postpartum asphyxia. The disadvantages of this method are due to the relative complexity of the technique, the discontinuous and invasive nature of the method, and the few contraindications to its use (1).

1.1.6.2. Scalp lactates

This 2nd-line method is as reliable as scalp pH, but with higher specificity for metabolic acidosis. The sampling technique is simpler than that of scalp pH. The amount of blood required is smaller, and the failure rate is lower. Nevertheless, this method does not improve neonatal status, and there are no studies to show a reduction in obstetric interventions (1).

1.1.6.3. Fetal pulse oximetry

I Oximetry is a technique that continuously monitors intrapartum fetal oxygen saturation. It was first tested in the late 1990's. The main drawback of oximetry is signal loss, particularly during uterine contractions and fetal head advancement. This invasive procedure involves transvaginal placement of sensors on the fetal cheek or temple after rupture of the membranes (14). This technique was virtually abandoned in the mid-2000s; most studies agree that the addition of fetal pulse oximetry does not reduce overall caesarean section rates (11,15).

1.1.6.4. Fetal electrocardiogram (ECG) with computerized ST-segment analysis

This is an invasive technique used in conjunction with ERCF. It involves placing an electrode on the scalp after the membrane has ruptured. The fetal

ECG can be monitored during labor while recording fetal heart rate and uterine activity.

To compare the efficacy of ERCF combined with ST analysis with cardiotocography alone during labor, a systematic review and meta-analysis of six of randomized controlled trials (16), which included 26,529 women in labor, were analyzed. Concluded that the use of ST-segment analysis during labor in addition to standard cardiotocography does not improve perinatal outcomes, nor does it reduce the rate of cesarean deliveries. This technique is therefore not recommended in clinical practice, and warrants further investigation (11).

References

1. Text of recommendations. J Gynécologie Obstétrique Biol Reprod . févr 2008 ;37(1):S101-7.
2. Houfflin-Debarge V, Closset E, Deruelle P. Surveillance du travail dans les situations à risque. J Gynécologie Obstétrique Biol Reprod [Internet]. Feb 2008;37(1):S81-92.
3. M. J. The partograph: A labour management tool or a midwifery record? Int J Nurs Midwifery . Dec 31, 2013;5(8):145-53.6
4. Anokye R, Acheampong E, Anokye J, Budu-Ainooson A, Amekudzie E, Owusu I, et al. Use and completion of partograph during labour is associated with a reduced incidence of birth asphyxia: a retrospective study at a peri-urban setting in Ghana. J Health Popul Nutr. May 16, 2019 ;38.
5. Greenwood C, Lalchandani S, MacQuillan K, Sheil O, Murphy J, Impey L. Meconium passed in labor: how reassuring is clear amniotic fluid? Obstet Gynecol. Jul 2003;102(1):89-93.
6. Becker S, Solomayer E, Dogan C, Wallwiener D, Fehm T. Meconium-stained amniotic fluid--perinatal outcome and obstetrical management in a low-risk suburban population. Eur J Obstet Gynecol Reprod Biol. May 2007;132(1):46-50.
7. Maymon E, Chaim W, Furman B, Ghezzi F, Shoham Vardi I, Mazor M. Meconium stained amniotic fluid in very low risk pregnancies at term gestation. Eur J Obstet Gynecol Reprod Biol. Oct 1998;80(2):169-73.
8. Mundhra R, Agarwal M. Fetal outcome in meconium stained deliveries. J Clin Diagn Res JCDR. Dec 2013;7(12):2874-6.
9. De Souza A, Minebois H, Luc A, Choserot M, Bertholdt C, Morel O, et al. Stained or meconium amniotic fluid: should they modify our obstetrical management? Gynécologie Obstétrique Fertil Sénologie. janv 2018;46(1):28-33.
10. Visser GH, Ayres-de-Campos D, FIGO Intrapartum Fetal Monitoring Expert Consensus Panel. FIGO consensus guidelines on intrapartum fetal monitoring: Adjunctive technologies. Int J Gynaecol Obstet Off Organ Int Fed Gynaecol Obstet. oct 2015;131(1):25-9
11. Levy G, Bednarek N, Gabriel R. E. EM-Consulte. Per partum fetal asphyxia and fetal conditions not reassuring.
12. Macones GA, Hankins GDV, Spong CY, Hauth J, Moore T. The 2008 National Institute of Child Health and Human Development workshop report on electronic fetal monitoring: update on definitions, interpretation, and research guidelines. Obstet Gynecol. Sept 2008;112(3):661-6.

13. Carbonne B, Nguyen A. Fetal monitoring by scalp pH and lactate measurement during labor. J Gynécologie Obstétrique Biol Reprod . févr 2008 ;37(1):S65-71.

14. Vayssière C, David E, Meyer N, Haberstich R, Sebahoun V, Roth E, et al. A French randomized controlled trial of ST-segment analysis in a population with abnormal Cardiotocograms during labor. Am J Obstet Gynecol. Sept 2007;197(3):299.e1-6.

15. East CE, Begg L, Colditz PB, Lau R. Fetal pulse oximetry for fetal assessment in labour. Cochrane Database Syst Rev. 7 Oct 2014 ;2014(10).

16. Saccone G, Schuit E, Amer-Wâhlin I, Xodo S, Berghella V. Electrocardiogram ST Analysis During Labor: A Systematic Review and Meta-analysis of Randomized Controlled Trials. Obstet Gynecol. janv 2016;127(1):127-35.

1.2. Diagnosis after birth

1.2.1. Clinical diagnosis

1.2.1.1. Apgar score

The Apgar score was first described in 1950 by American anesthetist Virginia Apgar. It is the oldest and most commonly used assessment tool for evaluating the newborn immediately after delivery (1).

It corresponds to the recording of five parameters: heart and respiratory rates, tone, coloration and reactivity. It is scored from 0-10, with each item assigned a score of 0, 1 or 2, and the total gives the final score. A score of 7 or more suggests a favorable outcome for the newborn **(Table 1)**.

Table 1: Apgar score

PARAMETERS	0	1	2
Heartbeats	Absent	Less than 100 per minute	More than 100 per minute
Breathing movements	Absent	Slow, irregular	Regular, vigorous, with cry
Muscle tone	Null, flaccid	Weak: slight bending of extremities	Quadriflexion, active movements
Reactivity to stimulation	Null	Weak; slight movement,	Vive: screaming, coughing

		grimace	
Color	Overall blue or pale	Pink body, blue tips	Totally pink

The Apgar score provided a quantitative expression of the immediate postnatal status of newborns, and was designed to serve as a guide for assessing the need for resuscitation. On the other hand, the Apgar score assigned during resuscitation and intubation does not provide an accurate assessment of the neonate's condition.

It is important to recognize the limitations of the Apgar score. It is an expression of the infant's physiological state at a given time, which includes subjective elements. Many factors can influence the Apgar score, including maternal sedation or anesthesia, congenital malformations, gestational age, trauma and inter-observer variability.

Because of these conditions, the Apgar score alone cannot be considered as evidence or consequence of asphyxia (2).

What's more, the score awarded during resuscitation does not reflect the real condition of these newborns. The Apgar score assigned during resuscitation is called the "assisted Apgar score" and is not equivalent to that assigned to a spontaneously breathing infant. In other words, it would be misleading to assign a "2" for respirations to an intubated newborn who has no spontaneous breathing at 5 minutes of age and is ventilated at 30 breaths per minute. To correctly describe these newborns, the American Academy of Pediatrics (AAP) and the American College of Obstetricians and Gynecologists (2) have proposed an expanded Apgar score form that takes into account concomitant resuscitation interventions. Several studies have attempted to verify the impact of a low Apgar score at 5 minutes on mortality.Casey et al (3) in a retrospective analysis of 132,228 full-term babies, the mortality rate was 244 per 1,000 for newborns with five-minute Apgar scores of 0 to 3, compared with 0.2 per 1,000 for those with a five-minute Apgar score of 7 to 10; thus, an Apgar score at 5ème minutes remained strongly predictive of neonatal morbidity and mortality.

Another study, based on several North American registries of births and deaths, concluded that newborns with an Apgar score at five minutes of life of less than 3 had significantly higher neonatal and postnatal mortality rates, regardless of term, than those with higher scores. Moreover, if the score was ≥ 7, mortality decreased progressively with increasing gestational age (4).

1.2.1.2. Clinical examination of the newborn

A neurological examination should be carried out rapidly in the delivery room, to look for signs of encephalopathy in the newborn. This is an essential part of the neonatal assessment. The clinical picture of asphyxia in term newborns may present with the following symptoms:

- **Damage to the central nervous system**

These include coma, lethargy, hyporeactivity, respiratory depression, feeding difficulties, decreased motility, weak or absent cry, diminished or abolished primary reflexes, and active or passive hypotonia.

- **Neurovegetative disorders**

- sympathetic signs: tachycardia, mydriasis, scarcity of secretions
- parasympathetic signs: bradycardia, miosis, abundant secretions, diarrhea with increased intestinal peristalsis, bronchial obstruction due to

hypersecretion, bronchospasm

- **Hyperexcitability**

High-pitched, excessive crying, permanent hyperactivity, osteotendinous reflexes and vivid archaic reflexes.

- **Intracranial hypertension**

It is characterized by: increased cranial perimeter (CP), fontanel tension, suture disjunction, signs of cerebral edema such as: bradycardia, apneas, hypertonia of the neck extensors, opisthotonos.

The presence of convulsive activity during the first hours of life is one of the typical manifestations of CNS damage due to asphyxia.

A neurological examination should be carried out rapidly in the delivery room, to look for signs of encephalopathy in the newborn. It is an essential part of the neonatal assessment.

Clinical assessment of the severity of neurological damage is usually based on the Sarnat and Sarnat classification (5), which has prognostic value.

Grade I: Mild encephalopathy

> Irritability, hyperexcitability, normal muscle tone, normal or increased reflexes, ankle tremor on stimulation, absence of seizures.

> These signs are often transient, disappearing within 48 hours.

- **Grade II: Moderate encephalopathy**

Lethargy, disturbed consciousness, reduced spontaneous movements, proximal muscle weakness, reduced archaic reflexes, clinical or subclinical seizures.

- **Grade III: Severe encephalopathy**

  Coma or stupor, major hypotonia, absence of archaic reflexes, frequent and difficult-to-control convulsive seizures.

Grade I is associated with a good prognosis with no sequelae. Grade II is associated with an intermediate prognosis: 40 to 60% of sequelae. Grade III is associated with a very unfavorable prognosis, with close to 100% death or serious sequelae (6).

Another clinical score used for the clinical assessment of AIA is the Thompson score, described in 1996, based on the longitudinal clinical assessment of 9 signs. Each sign is scored from 0 to 3, and the total score for each day is calculated. It enables early identification of children with a poor prognosis (7).

1.2.1.3. Convulsions

Anoxic-ischemic encephalopathy is the most frequent cause of neonatal seizures. Seizures generally occur within two days of birth, and those observed before 6 hours should raise suspicion of a previous aggression in utero (8).

They can take one of the following forms:

- ***Frustrating forms***: with clonies (chin, eyelids, diaphragm), chewing and pedaling movements, apneas;

- ***Tonic seizures***: stiff newborns, in opisthotonos, with contracture and extension of the limbs;

- ***Multi-focal clonic seizures***: accompanied by bursts of clonia migrating from one limb to another;

- ***Focal seizures***: focal clonus remains localized;

- ***Myoclonic convulsions (rare)***: these are irregular jerks in flexion of a lower or upper limb, of variable duration.

Seizures increase the cerebral metabolic load, trigger the release of excitatory neurotransmitters and cause cardiorespiratory instability, exacerbating the condition of neurons.

Neonatal seizures are usually diagnosed by clinical observation, but this can be very difficult. The semiology of seizures in neonates can be subtle, and dystonic movements or brainstem reactions may be mistaken for seizures. Both over- and under-interpretation have been reported. Standard video EEG has been considered ideal for the accurate diagnosis of neonatal epileptic seizures, but is not feasible in most neonatal departments due to lack of availability (9).

In a study comparing clinical observations and video electroencephalography (EEG), two-thirds of clinical manifestations were either unrecognized or misinterpreted by experienced neonatal staff (10).

There are four possible scenarios that can lead to a diagnosis of neonatal seizures (9):

1. **Clinical seizures with confirmed electrical abnormalities on EEG**: correlate with clinical seizures, and are directly responsible for the clinical instability observed. (Hemodynamic instability, respiratory problems, decreased level of consciousness).
2. **Clinical seizures with electrographic abnormalities but no clinical instability**

3. **No clinically identifiable seizures, but apparent electro-graphic abnormalities**

4. **Clinical seizures without any electro-graphic abnormalities**: could result from misdiagnosis of clinical seizures or could be true clinical seizures that do not result in electrical abnormalities on the EEG

1.2.2. Paraclinical diagnosis

1.2.2.1. Blood gas in cord blood

Blood gas analysis is the cornerstone of diagnosis, enabling us to diagnose or rule out perinatal asphyxia (11).

1.2.2.1.1. The different measures

Blood gas analysis provides the following values: pH, pCO_2 , pO_2 , bicarbonates and base deficit. However, only pH, base deficit and pCO2 are useful for confirming the presence and/or type of acidosis. To distinguish respiratory from metabolic acidosis, base deficit (>12mmol/L) or lactate (>8mmol/L) values must be recorded (12,13).

1.2.2.1.2. Sampling method

Acid-base balance is measured in the umbilical artery as soon as possible, at less than one hour after birth. Samples should be taken from the umbilical artery with a heparinized syringe, reflecting the aci- dobasic state of the fetus, whereas venous samples from the placenta better reflect the quality of placental exchange.

The blood sample should be kept at room temperature for a maximum of one hour. If analysis cannot be performed within one hour of birth, the sample can be kept on ice to prevent the leukocytes that remain active from consuming large quantities of oxygen and releasing carbon dioxide (14).

1.2.2.1.3. Standards

The normal fetus has an arterial pH close to 7.35. There is a physiological decrease during labor, and the normal value of umbilical arterial pH is 7.24 ± 0.07. A pH below 7.15 defines neonatal acidosis (12). Normal cord blood gas values are shown in **Table 2**.

Table 1: Normal and limit values for cord artery blood gases at birth

Parameters	Typical values (5-95)^{cile}	Pathological thresholds	Sequels
pH	7,15-7,4	< 7,15	< 7,00
pO2 (mmHg)	8-30	< 8	
PCO2 (mm Hg)	55	> 65	-
Base deficit (Meq/l)	2,7 à 4,9	> 8	>12
Lactates (mmol/l)	1-8	> 5	-

1.2.2.1.4. Indications

According to the Collège National des Gynécologues et Obstétriciens Français (CNGOF), it is advisable to systematically perform gasometry at the cord (arterial and, if possible, venous). If it is not possible to perform it systematically, it is recommended to do so in the event of RCF anomalies (professional agreement)(^).

-*The American College of Obstetricians and Gynecologists (ACOG)* and the American Academy of Pediatrics (AAP) recommend it in cases of low Apgar score at 5 minutes, intrauterine growth retardation, abnormal fetal heart rate, maternal thyroid disease, intrapartum fever and multiple pregnancy (15,16).

1.2.2.2. Measuring lactates in cord blood

Lactate is a product of glucose breakdown during anaerobic metabolism in the event of asphyxia. Its presence confirms the metabolic origin of acidosis. Measured with the same equipment as for scalp lactate. Despite its lower cost, cord lactate measurement is not considered equivalent to conventional gasometry (15).

1.2.2.3. Other biomarkers

1.2.2.3.1. Interleukins

Interleukins (ILs), known to be one of the first inflammatory responses to infection, are involved in the biochemical pathways leading to ischemic and hypoxic lesions during perinatal asphyxia.

Recent studies have focused on inflammatory cytokines such as IL-1β, IL6 and IL8 for the early diagnosis of brain damage. The role of inflammation in neonatal central nervous system (CNS) injury and the role of cytokines as mediators of injury have been identified. The identification of biochemical markers such as interleukins (ILs) can be useful for the early diagnosis of asphyxia, providing better care and improving prognosis. The combination of IL6 and IL-1β can be used as a powerful marker for the early diagnosis of perinatal asphyxia (17,18).

1.2.2.3.2. Biomarkers

Various biomarkers of brain injury in blood, urine and CSF have been proposed, including ,calcium-binding protein B (S100B), glial fibrillary acidic protein (GFAP), ubiquitin carboxyl-terminal hydrolase L1 (UCH-L1), brain band creatine kinase, neuron-specific enolase (NSE), malodialdehyde and pro-inflammatory cytokines ; All these markers of asphyxia have been studied previously and may hold promise for measuring the severity of ischemic hypoxic injury. They can be used to guide interventions, assess the effects of treatment and provide prognostic information to parents. At present, the precise sensitivity is not yet known (19,20).

1.2.2.4. Standard electroencephalogram (EEG)

Electroencephalography (EEG) remains a valuable aid in the management of full-term newborns presenting with asphyxia.

It is a reproducible, non-traumatic means of cerebral exploration that can be performed at the patient's bedside. It continues to have relevant and early diagnostic and predictive value in neonates (21).

- **Diagnostic interest** :

  Identification of abnormal EEG aspects, so as not to overlook another etiology of neonatal encephalopathy.

- **Prognostic interest:**

  The prognostic value of electroencephalography (EEG) in term newborns with EAI has been well demonstrated using recordings obtained between days 2 and 7. It is based on the estimation of the degree of severity, which may be related to :

  -**EEG types**: normal, pejorative (inactive, paroxysmal, poor in theta waves) or "intermediate" (discontinuous type A or B, rapid hyperactivity) (22)

  - **Time to normalization**: severe abnormalities recorded before 12 hours of birth may be rapidly reversible, and the EEG has no prognostic value in this context. However, such abnormalities may be an indication for neuroprotective treatment (23).

When to register?

The first tracing should be carried out between 12 and 48 hours of life (prolonged or continuous), and controls should be carried out on the fourth and eighth days of life, or even earlier, depending on clinical symptoms and the results of the first EEG.

From the first week of life, check-ups are recommended according to the child's electro-clinical development (24).

The analysis of the background traces concerns: morphology according to the Dreyfus-Brisac classification (22), which allows classification into four stages:

- **Type 1**: normal trace or minor anomalies (excess theta rhythms, temporal spikes, moderate asymmetry)
- **Type 2** : pathological slow wave pattern in term newborns: continuous delta-frequency activity (0.5-1.5 Hz), diffuse, low amplitude (less than 50 μV), present in both wakefulness and sleep, with little reactivity.
- **Type 3A and 3B**: discontinuous routes with type A or B activity representing more than 50% of the route:

→ type 3A: The duration of each puff is between 10 and 30 s and includes physiological elements, frontal notches separated by weakly volted intervals of amplitude less than 10 μV and less than 10 s.

→ type 3B: puffs are made up of theta elements whose duration varies from 10 to 30 s and amplitude from 30 to 50 μV and are separated by intervals of amplitude less than 10 μV, and duration less than 10 s. It has no physiological graphoelement or spatiotemporal organization, and is not very labile.

- **Type 4**: very pathological trace, inactive poor plus theta rhythm, or paroxysmal.

1.2.2.5. Amplitude EEG

The use of amplitude-integrated electroencephalography (aEEG) has become standard practice in most neonatal units in developed countries, and is part of the standard protocol for the management of EAI. The use and interpretation of aEEG in clinical practice is straightforward and has been reported to have high specificity and low sensitivity.

This method offers the possibility of improved diagnosis of electrographic seizures, with or without clinical seizures (25).

appeared in adult anesthesia at the end of the 1960s. Cerebral monitoring of vulnerable newborns was developed in the 1980s for use in anoxic-ischemic situations in full-term neonates.

This is a device designed to "monitor" the electroencephalographic trace over long periods ranging from a few hours to a few days.

Recording is made using two electrodes on the scalp; the signal is usually collected in a single lead from a pair of electrodes placed on the parietal region, amplified and filtered, with only frequencies between 2 and 15 Hz retained (26).

Interpretation

Several classifications exist for interpreting an aEEG, one of the most accessible being that described by al Naqeeb et al (27).

The basic elements are the amplitude, which corresponds globally to the background trace of the standard EEG, and the values of the lower and upper limits of the band produced by the aEEG recording. The different types are shown in **Fig. 2** :

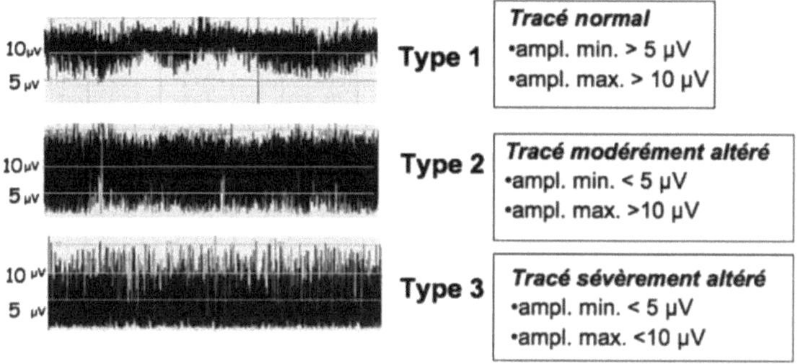

Figure 1: *Types of amplitude EEG (23)*

Continuous monitoring can detect sub-clinical seizures, for example in at-risk newborns, whose sedation for mechanical ventilation may mask these events. It also provides information on the efficacy of antiepileptic treatment.

It must be validated by performing a standard EEG, because of the possibility of artifacts or impedance errors. It is a monitoring tool used in neuroprotection protocols (26).

1.2.2.6. X-ray examinations

1.2.2.6.1. Trans-fontanelle ultrasound (TFE)

Cranial or transfontanellar ultrasound relies on the reflection of ultrasound waves on tissues to provide images. It remains the most commonly used neuroimaging technique in neonatal intensive care units, as it is inexpensive, portable, involves no radiation exposure and requires no special preparation.

ETF may be the only imaging technique available when a newborn is clinically unstable. It can be performed even for neonates undergoing invasive ventilation (28).

Despite these advantages, this technique has certain limitations: incomplete peripheral exploration, difficulty in studying the cortex and structures of the posterior fossa, and lack of sensitivity in determining the extent of cerebral lesions, even in cases of severe encephalopathy and especially in the first 24 hours of life. When performed, it usually reveals diffuse hyperechogenicity of the cerebral cortex and subcortical white matter, lenticular nuclei and thalamus (29).

It allows us to exclude certain causes of neonatal encephalopathy, antenatal lesions and major brain damage (16).

1.2.2.6.2. Computed tomography (CT) of the brain

It offers a number of advantages, including quantitative measurement of tissue diffusivity and high sensitivity for the detection of acute hemorrhage. These advantages are useful for assessing acute brain pathology, particularly in the context of traumatic brain injury (16). This technique can differentiate hyperdense hemorrhagic lesions from hypodense ischemic lesions. Sometimes, it is difficult to assess the extent of pathological (ischemic) hypodensity in areas of physiological hypodensity (parenchymal immaturity).

Subcortical hypoxia-ischemia lesions present as hypodensity when extensive. It reflects diffuse cytotoxic cerebral edema and is a poor prognostic factor (28).

1.2.2.6. 3. Magnetic resonance imaging

In full-term newborns, MRI has become the preferred brain imaging modality due to its superior sensitivity and specificity for detecting and quantifying brain abnormalities, and because it does not expose newborns to ionizing radiation (30).

Magnetic resonance imaging is an excellent prognostic tool. It has the major advantage of being the most comprehensive method for assessing macrostructural and microstructural cerebral and vascular anatomy. It is the reference examination in EAI. It will enable us to better define the nature and extent of cerebral lesions in neonatal encephalopathy. The main disadvantage of MRI is the need to transport highly unstable neonates out of ICUs (16).

Various techniques are used in EAI

- **Conventional MRI**

It does not allow early identification of cerebral lesions, due to edema. Brain scan, which interferes with the interpretation of the white matter signal. For this reason, it is recommended to perform it later, between D7 and D10 of life (28).

- **Diffusion MRI**

This technique can be used to determine the presence of early cytotoxic edema in the event of tissue ischemia, through the reduction of extracellular spaces resulting in a decrease in the spontaneous diffusion of water molecules. It enables early lesions to be detected, between the first and fourth day after birth, before the appearance of abnormalities on conventional sequences (31).

- **Other MRI techniques**

Magnetic resonance spectroscopy provides complementary metabolic information and has also proved to be a reliable prognostic biomarker.

Other advanced MRI techniques, including diffusion tensor imaging and arterial spin labeling, are currently being used to gain further insight into the etiology and prognosis of brain lesions (30).

Different types of lesions

The extent and location of brain damage in newborns with perinatal asphyxia depend on the severity, timing and duration of the hypoxic-ischemic event, in addition to the maturation of the brain at the time of the event.
Three main types of lesions can be distinguished in infants with HIE **(Figure 3)**:

- **Lesions of the basal ganglia and thalamus**: lesions associated with motor neurodevelopment disorders, including cerebral palsy (32).
- **White matter lesions**: this type of lesion is often not very serious and lasts only a short time. However, follow-up is necessary, given the risk of long-term cognitive impairment (33).
- **Near-total or global lesions**: diffuse lesions both in the UCS and in the white matter. This is the case in severe asphyxia, where the patient dies before MRI can be performed.

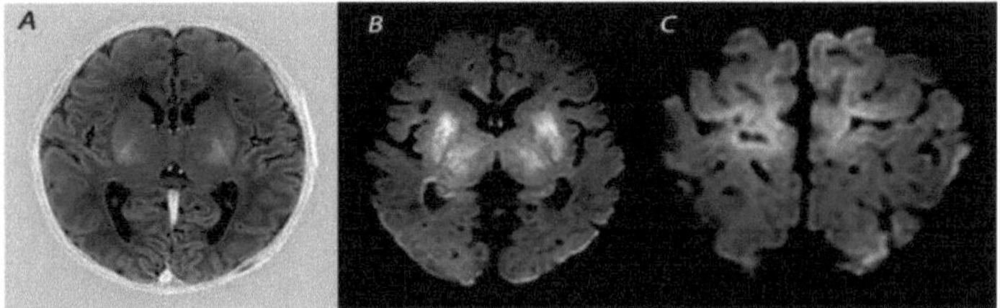

Basal ganglia involvement: (A) internal capsule, (B) and (C) thalamus

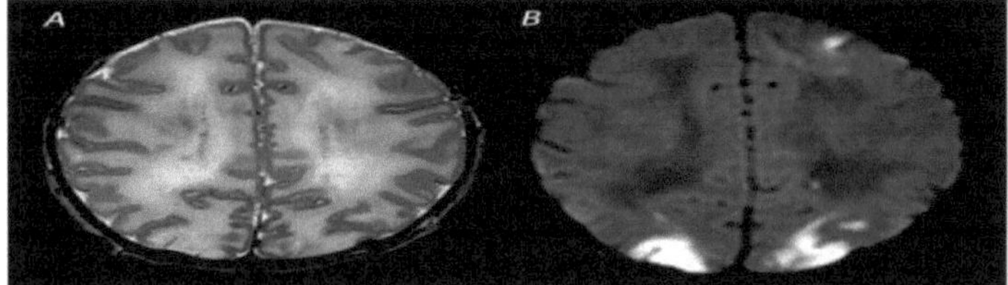

White matter involvement:(A) and(B) occipital lobes and left frontal lobe

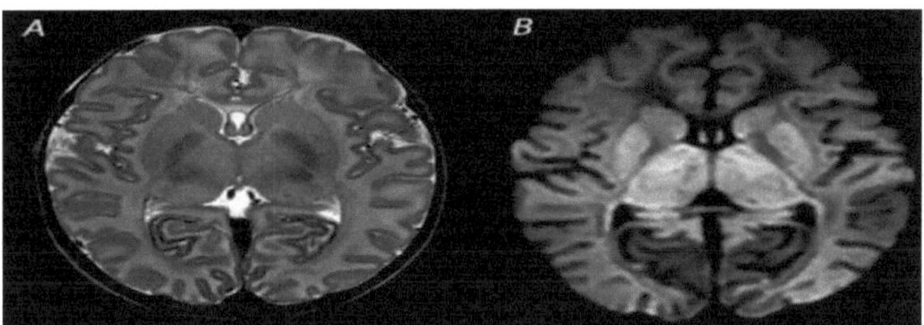

Global damage:(A) and (B) white matter, UCS, brainstem and cerebellum

Figure 2: *Appearance of MRI lesions* ***(33)***

References

1. Apgar V. A proposal for a new method of evaluation of the newborn infant. Curr Res Anesth Analg. August 1953;32(4):260-7.

2. American Academy of Pediatrics, Committee on Fetus and Newborn, American College of Obstetricians and Gynecologists, Committee on Obstetric Practice. The Apgar Score. Pediatrics. 1 Apr 2006 ;117(4):1444-7.

3. Casey BM, McIntire DD, Leveno KJ. The Continuing Value of the Apgar Score for the Assessment of Newborn Infants. N Engl J Med [Internet]. Feb 15, 2001 [cited Feb 20, 2022];344(7):467-71.

4. Li F, Wu T, Lei X, Zhang H, Mao M, Zhang J. The Apgar Score and Infant Mortality. Gong Y, editor. PLoS ONE 29 Jul 2013 ;8(7):e69072.

5. Sarnat HB, Sarnat MS. Neonatal encephalopathy following fetal distress. A clinical and electroencephalographic study. Arch Neurol. Oct 1976;33(10):696-705.

6. Zupan Simunek V. Definition of intrapartum asphyxia and consequences for outcome.

Rev Sage-Femme . mai 2008 ;7(2):79-86

7. Thompson CM, Puterman AS, Linley LL, Hann FM, van der Elst CW, Molteno CD, et al. The value of a scoring system for hypoxic ischaemic encephalopathy in predicting neurodevelopmental outcome. Acta Paediatr Oslo Nor 1992. July 1997;86(7):757-61.

8. Martinello K, Hart AR, Yap S, Mitra S, Robertson NJ. Management and investigation of neonatal encephalopathy: 2017 update. Arch Dis Child Fetal Neonatal Ed [Internet]. jul 2017;102(4):F346-58.

9. Shetty J. Neonatal seizures in hypoxic-ischaemic encephalopathy - risks and benefits of anticonvulsant therapy. Dev Med Child Neurol . Apr 2015 ;57:40-3.

10. Murray DM, Boylan GB, Ali I, Ryan CA, Murphy BP, Connolly S. Defining the gap between electrographic seizure burden, clinical expression and staff recognition of neonatal seizures. Arch Dis Child - Fetal Neonatal Ed [Internet]. May 1, 2008 [cited March 26, 2023];93(3):F187-91.

11. Carbonne B, Nguyen A. Fetal monitoring by scalp pH and lactate measurement during labor. J Gynécologie Obstétrique Biol Reprod . févr 2008 ;37(1):S65-71.

12. Leboucher B, Huetz N, Gascoin G. Perinatal biology: the pediatrician's point of view. Rev Francoph Lab [Internet]. march 2015 ;2015(470):25-31.

13. LANGER.B, LECOINTRE.A.Comme.Comment interpréter les gaz du sang au cordon ombilical ?réalités pédiatriques # 192_Mars 2015].

14. Thorp JA, Rushing RS. Umbilical cord blood gas analysis. Obstet Gynecol Clin North Am. Dec 1999;26(4):695-709.

15. Text of recommendations. J Gynécologie Obstétrique Biol Reprod . févr 2008

;37(1):S101-7.

16. Executive summary: Neonatal encephalopathy and neurologic outcome, second edition. Report of the American College of Obstetricians and Gynecologists' Task Force on Neonatal Encephalopathy. Obstet Gynecol. 2014 Apr;123(4):896-901

17. Boskabadi H, Afshari JT, Ghayour-Mobarhan M, Maamouri G, Shakeri MT, Sahebkar A, et al. Association between serum interleukin-6 levels and severity of perinatal asphyxia. Asian Biomed. 2010 ;4(1):79-85.

18. Boskabadi H, Moradi A, Zakerihamidi M. Interleukins in diagnosis of perinatal asphyxia: A systematic review. Int J Reprod Biomed ;17(5):303-14

19. Tekgul H, Yalaz M, Kutukculer N, Ozbek S, Kose T, Akisu M, et al. Value of biochemical markers for outcome in term infants with asphyxia. Pediatr Neurol . nov 2004 ;31(5):326-32.

20. Ramaswamy V, Horton J, Vandermeer B, Buscemi N, Miller S, Yager J. Systematic Review of Biomarkers of Brain Injury in Term Neonatal Encephalopathy. Pediatr Neurol . March 2009 ;40(3):215-26.

21. André-Obadia N, Sauleau P, Cheliout-Heraut F, Convers P, Debs R, Eisermann M, et al. French recommendations on electroencephalogram. Neurophysiol Clin Neurophysiol Dec 2014;44(6):515-612.

22. Gire C, Nicaise C, Roussel M, Soula F, Girard N, Somma-Mauvais H, et al. Hypoxoischemic encephalopathy of the term newborn. Contribution of electroencephalogram and MRI or CT to prognostic evaluation. À propos de 26 observationsNeurophysiol Clin 2000 ; 30 : 97-107.

23. Pressler RM, Boylan GB, Morton M, Binnie CD, Rennie JM. Early serial EEG in hypoxic ischaemic encephalopathy. Clin Neurophysiol Jan 2001;112(1):31-7.

24. Lamblin MD, André M, Auzoux M, Bednarek N, Bour F, Charollais A, et al. Indications for electroencephalogram in the neonatal period. Arch Pédiatrie . juill 2004;11(7):829-33.

25. Shetty J. Neonatal seizures in hypoxic-ischaemic encephalopathy - risks and benefits of anticonvulsant therapy. Dev Med Child Neurol . Apr 2015 ;57:40-3.

26. Bednarek N, Delebarre G, Saad S, Loron G, Mezguiche F, Morville P. Amplitude EEG: description, applications, advantages and disadvantages. Arch Pediatrie . August 2008;15(8):1326-31.

27. al Naqeeb N, Edwards AD, Cowan FM, Azzopardi D. Assessment of Neonatal Encephalopathy by Amplitude-integrated Electroencephalography. Pediatrics . June 1, 1999;103(6):1263-71.

28. Aloui-Kasbi N, Allani H, Mrad S, Bellagha I, Hammou A. Perinatal asphyxia and brain imaging. J Pédiatrie Puériculture . oct 2003 ;16(6):312-5.

29. Bano S, Chaudhary V, Garga U. Neonatal hypoxic-ischemic encephalopathy: A radiological review. J Pediatr Neurosci. 2017 ;12(1):1.

30. Sorokan ST, Jefferies AL, Miller SP. Brain imaging of the term newborn.

Paediatr Child Health. 2018;23(5):329-35.

31. Meyer-Witte S, Brissaud O, Brun M, Lamireau D, Bordessoules M, Chateil JF. Prognostic contribution of cerebral magnetic resonance in hypoxic-ischemic encephalopathy of the term newborn: imaging score, spectroscopy. Study of 26 cases. Arch Pediatrics. Jan 2008 ;15(1):9-23.

32. Martinez-Biarge M, Diez-Sebastian J, Kapellou O, Gindner D, Allsop JM, Rutherford MA, et al. Predicting motor outcome and death in term hypoxic-ischemic encephalopathy. Neurology . June 14, 2011 ;76(24):2055-61.

33. *Parmentier CEJ, de Vries LS, Groenendaal F. Magnetic Resonance Imaging in (Near-)Term* Infants with Hypoxic-Ischemic Encephalopathy. Diagnostics. March 6, 2022
;12(3):645.

Chapter 4

1. Etiological factors

Factors leading to interruption of blood flow in APN are related to labor, the fetus, the adnexa, the maternal condition, iatrogenic substances or behavioral etiological factors (1,2,3,4).

1.1. Maternal causes

1.1.1. Chronic conditions

Placental lesions and altered vascularization due to preeclampsia, diabetes, prolonged pregnancy; anemia and cardio-respiratory insufficiency: these pathologies lead to maternal hypoxia, which can affect fetal oxygenation.

1.1.2. Acute pathologies

A sudden drop in placental perfusion, either as a result of hypertonia in response to HRP, hemorrhagic shock, or the Poseiro effect, i.e. the change in uterine position that accompanies uterine contraction, leading to compression of the aorta during dorsal decubitus. This effect results in reduced utero-placental blood supply and maternal discomfort. Other emergencies such as convulsions, suffocating pneumothorax and abdominal trauma can also explain fetal hypoxia.

1.2. Iatrogenic causes

The role of iatrogenesis is not negligible in the genesis of asphyxia. Indeed, several drugs are incriminated:

- Oxytocics act through hyperkinesia or hypertonia when used inappropriately
- Antispasmodics and analgesics can be harmful when injected in late labor, as they depress the respiratory centers of the fetus and can

result in asphyxia.

- Epidural analgesia or excessive use of antihypertensive drugs can cause iatrogenic hypotension and thus acute quantitative insufficiency of maternal oxygenation.
- General anesthetics act by depressing maternal respiratory centers.

1.3. Work-related causes

These anomalies affect either uterine contraction (UC) or the duration of labor.

1.3.1. CU anomalies

It can be either a frequency anomaly or an intensity anomaly of the UC. There are two types:

- **Frequency hyperkinesia**: CUs exceed 5 CU/10min, which reduces interphasic relaxation time.
- **Intensity hyperkinesia**: the UC is greater and more prolonged, with an intensity greater than 60mmHg at the start and 80mmHg at the end of labor.
- **Hypertonia:** the basic tone is greater than 11mmHg at the beginning and 18mmHg at the end of labor, with no interphasic relaxation. Hyperkinesia often reflects the uterus' struggle against an obstacle, as is the case in fetal-pelvic disproportion. Hypertonia is seen in acute accidents such as retroplacental hematoma, and in mechanical dystocia, where it is the final stage before uterine rupture.

1.3.2. Working time anomalies

All forms of dystocia, especially dynamic dystocia, can be the cause of abnormally prolonged labor.

They can lead to fetal distress, which should be anticipated and investigated in such circumstances. Labor that lasts too long can deplete the oxygen supply in the inter-ventricular chamber. It can also be a source of maternal overwork, with ventilation disorders: hypocapnia and major respiratory alkalosis.

These ventilation anomalies lead to a reduction in utero-placental flow and thus to fetal hypoxia.

The duration of the expulsion phase is also important, as the pH drops by : - 0.003 U/min during head descent to full dilatation; - 0.04 U/min during head expulsion and - 0.14 U/min during trunk expulsion. With this in mind, we recommend limiting these phases to 30min, 2min 30s and 40s respectively.

1.4. Fetal causes

Many cases of perinatal asphyxia occur when the fetus is in a precarious state:

- **Hypotrophy:** whether related to maternal complications or not, hypotrophy represents a situation at risk of asphyxia.
- **Macrosomia:** is also a situation at risk of FH, due to the particular fragility of macrosomia to hypoglycemia in the peri- and postpartum period and the high risk of shoulder dystocia.
- **Post-maturity**: by placental alterations with reduction in the surface area of the placenta's exchange membrane

- **Twin pregnancies**: exhaustion of transfusion recipients

1.5. Annex factors

1.5.1. Placental alterations

Acute retroplacental hematoma occurs in the context of pre-eclampsia or violent trauma. It is a source of severe FAS, which progresses more or less rapidly to BCF negativation, depending on the extent and location of the hematoma.

Other placental alterations are often the cause of APN: infarction, chorioangioma, placental villous hypotrophy, placental insufficiency during prolonged pregnancy, edema during diabetes or alloimmunization.

1.5.2. Funicular anomalies

Perinatal asphyxia may be related to a funicular anomaly involving cord compression or stretching. These cord position anomalies are: procubitus, procidence, laterocidence, tight circular, knot, sling, shortness of cord, velamentous insertion of cord: which can be the cause of lightning fetal hemorrhage through rupture of a previa vessel, Benkiser's hemorrhage.

1.5.3. Ovular factors

Oligohydramnios can cause funicular compression during uterine contractions. Placenta previa can lead to sudden hypotension as a result of hemorrhagic shock (retroplacental hematoma).

1.6. Social factors

Smoking, alcohol and poor socio-economic conditions....

2. Support

2.1. In the delivery room

2.1 .1. Resuscitation measures

At birth, effective cardiopulmonary resuscitation must be started as soon as possible to restore gas exchange and improve the cardiorespiratory status of asphyxiated newborns.

In 2000, standardized guidelines for neonatal resuscitation were drawn up by the International Liaison Task Force on Resuscitation (ILCOR). These guidelines are reviewed and revised on the basis of an evidence-based review, last updated in 2020, (5)

Recent recommendations give priority to positive pressure ventilation, with the use of a face mask or endotracheal tube, which is sufficient in most cases to restore hemodynamics and hematosis. Cardiac massage and the use of vasoactive drugs are necessary only after good ventilation has failed.

Air ventilation appears to be as effective as pure oxygen ventilation in most cases, and the toxic effects (free radical release) may be less.

2.1.1.1. Objectives and principles

The objectives of neonatal resuscitation are :

- Efficient ventilation
- Maintain a heart rate > 100 bpm
- Combating metabolic acidosis

Neonatal resuscitation follows the general principles of resuscitation according to the ABCD rule:

A: Airways: freeing the airways

B: Breathing: to induce breathing movements

C: Circulation: ensuring an efficient circulatory minimum

D: Drug: administer medicines and/or solutions.

2.1.1.2. Resuscitation diagram

Briefing:

- Define responsibilities, check equipment and plan stabilization or resuscitation.
- Roles and tasks need to be assigned; checklists are useful.
- Prepare the family if resuscitation is anticipated.

At each birth, the following characteristics must be assessed:

- ✓ Is the baby full term?
- ✓ Is the amniotic fluid clear?
- ✓ Is the child screaming or breathing?
- ✓ Does the child have good muscle tone?

If the answer to all 4 questions is "yes", the newborn does not require special care. This is not neonatal resuscitation. In this case, late cord clamping (beyond one minute) may be recommended.

If the answer to any of the 4 questions is "no", resuscitation procedures should be performed according to the following diagram

A. Preliminary stages

These 4 preliminary steps are essential before continuing any resuscitation. They should last no longer than 30 seconds.

1. Drying = preventing cooling.
2. Open the airway = position and aspirate.
3. Stimulate = trigger respiratory movements.
4. Assess the child's condition.

A. 1 Drying: Prevent cooling.

✓ Resuscitation room temperature >26°C

✓ Hot table, hot towels

Drying must be thorough and rapid, and damp linen must be disposed of immediately. The use of a cap and a polyethylene "survival blanket" is recommended;

A.2 Clearing the upper airways

✓ **Positioning the child** :

The newborn is placed in dorsal decubitus, with the neck in moderate extension and the head slightly sloping, to ensure a neutral position. Excessive flexion or extension of the head can obstruct the passage of air through the lower airways. To keep the child in this position, it may be necessary to use a block that raises the shoulders by 2-3 cm and lets the occiput rest on the mattress. This is particularly recommended when the volume of the head is increased by a serosanguineous bump or edema.

✓ **Suctioning the upper airway:**

Clearing the upper airway involves suctioning the mouth, pharynx and nostrils. Any violent or prolonged stimulation of the posterior wall of the pharynx in the first few minutes of life causes a vagal reflex responsible for severe bradycardia and/or apnea. For this reason, some authors no longer recommend systematic suctioning of newborns, even during resuscitation when the child is not obstructed.

- Suction pressure must be between -100 and -150 cm of water.
- Suction should be gentle and brief, and should always be performed when the probe is removed.
- It is essential to start with the mouth and then the nostrils, if necessary.
- To aspirate the mouth, we use a No. 10-gauge probe, inserted a maximum of 3 to 5 cm into the mouth. Suction is taken from the pharynx, under the tongue and inside the cheeks. Several passes may be necessary if suctioning is to be productive.
- To aspirate the nasal cavities, a n°8 or n°6 probe is used, inserted about 1cm successively into each nostril.

- It is advisable to make only one passage per nostril, as this could be traumatic and cause edema, leading to dyspnea or prolonged obstruction.

NB: Gastric aspiration is not a neonatal resuscitation procedure and should never be performed within the first 5 minutes of life, as it can lead to vagal malaise or bradycardia.

A.3 Stimulating

If drying and stimulation by upper airway suction are not sufficient to trigger spontaneous respiratory movements in the child, more specific tactile stimulation should be used.

The newborn is stimulated by gentle taps on the sole of the foot, "flicks" on the heel or firm, rapid back rubs.

These gestures should be rapid and brief, and may be continued, but should not delay the start of assisted ventilation if the child remains apneic.

NB: Holding a child upside down, shaking, spanking or spraying with cool liquid are now recognized as dangerous and completely unnecessary techniques.

A.4 Evaluate

The Apgar score is a good way of assessing the child's condition at 1, 5 and 10 minutes, but cannot be used to decide whether or not to resuscitate.

The child's assessment is based on the 3-point rule

C: cry, heart and color.

✓ Breathing

Breathing is assessed by the presence or absence of spontaneous movements of the thorax, as well as the frequency, amplitude, regularity and symmetry of thoracic expansion.

Irregular breathing, gasps or apneas are synonymous with inefficient ventilation.

✓ Heart rate

- It must be above 100 bpm.
- It is recommended that heart rate be assessed by auscultation of the heart rather than palpation of the base of the cord.
- Any change in heart rate reflects an improvement or deterioration in the child's condition.

✓ **Coloring**

Coloration is of little relevance in assessing the child's actual oxygenation, and is no longer used by the International Liaison Committee on Resuscitation (ILCOR) as a criterion for evaluating the effectiveness of resuscitation, since peripheral cyanosis is common in newborns. It often reflects circulatory slowdown in the extremities or cooling rather than oxygenation failure.

✓ **Oxygen saturation**

Oxygen saturation by pulse oximetry (SpO2) is an essential parameter, highlighted in the latest recommendations. It must be set up with the right hand, i.e. preductally (supraductally), and enables oxygen concentration to be adapted to the child's real needs.

B. Mask ventilation (Breathing)

B.1 Indications and contraindications

✓ **Indications**

- No effective spontaneous ventilation
- Apnea or gasps
- Heart rate < 100 bpm
- Persistent cyanosis.

B. 2 Air or oxygen?

- For full-term newborns, resuscitation should be started under ambient air.
- Oxygen is still indicated if first resuscitation is ineffective, and the

oxygen concentration must be adapted to the measurement of peripheral oxygen saturation (SpO2).

- The use of an air-oxygen mixer is recommended to allow greater reactivity in FiO2 variations.
- Ventilation technology
- The ventilatory rate is 40 cycles/min for a full-term newborn and 60 cycles/min for a premature infant.
- Insufflation time is about 3/4 of a second.

B. 3 Efficiency

Ventilation efficiency is assessed by :

- Symmetrical, regular thoracic movements
- Improved heart rate.

C. Tracheal intubation

C. 1 Indications

- Ineffective or inadequate mask ventilation
- Suspicion of congenital diaphragmatic hernia
- Bronchoaspiration in case of meconium inhalation
- Prolonged assisted ventilation

NB: The intubation manoeuvre should not exceed 20-30 seconds. If difficulties arise, the laryngoscope should be removed and mask ventilation resumed.

In the event of selective intubation, the probe should be removed by about 1cm and the symmetry of the vesicular murmur checked again by auscultation.

D. External cardiac massage (Circulation)

D. 1 Indication

A single indication: persistence of a heart rate < 60 bpm after 30 seconds of effective assisted ventilation with an adapted Fio2.

External cardiac massage should never be started immediately after birth, before the respiratory resuscitation maneuvers that are the priority in newborn resuscitation.

D.2. Techniques

- The aim of external cardiac massage is to ensure blood flow from the heart to the vital organs by rhythmic compression of the sternum, which presses the heart against the spine.
- Ventilation must obviously be continued, and two operators are required.
- Compressions should be made on the lower third of the sternum (below the bi-nipple line).
- Compressions and insufflations must be alternated to ensure effective action, at a rate of 3 compressions for 1 insufflation, i.e. 90 compressions and 30 insufflations per minute.
- Two techniques are possible, but it is the thumb technique with thorax impalement that is recommended today for its greater effectiveness.

D.3 Efficiency

- The effectiveness of MCE is assessed by the acceleration of the heart rate.

- It is checked every 30 seconds, as is breathing.

- Chest compressions should be maintained until the spontaneous heart rate is above 60 bpm.

E. Drugs

Drugs are rarely used in neonatal resuscitation. They are mainly administered to stimulate the heart, compensate for hypovolemia and improve tissue perfusion. Exceptionally, they are used to treat morphine-induced respiratory depression or correct aci- dobasic imbalance. Adrenaline is the first-line drug used in emergency resuscitation, and is indicated if heart rate < 60 bpm persists after 30 seconds of ECM combined with effective tube ventilation.

Intravenous (IV) administration via umbilical venous catheter (KTVO) is now the route recommended by ILCOR. Intra-tracheal administration remains an option, pending the availability of a venous approach.

Dosage: 1mg = 1mL ampoules are used, diluted with 9mL of 0.9% NaCl. The result is a diluted solution of 10mL = 1mg = 1000µg or 1ml = 100µg. IV: 10 to 30µgZkg = 0.1 to 0.3mL/kg. IT: 50 to 100µgZkg = 0.5 to 1 mL/kg.

Heart rate should increase rapidly to over 100bpm within 30 seconds of adrenaline administration. If this fails, the injection can be repeated every 3 to 5 minutes.

- After hypoxia-ischemia and primary energy failure, energy generation for ATP production depends on oxygen and glucose required for oxidative phosphorylation. Consequently, conditions that may delay recovery from the primary phase of brain injury, such as hypoxia, hypoglycemia, hypotension and anemia, must be corrected as soon as possible.

- Pending transfer to a hypothermia center, we recommend turning off the heating table to achieve passive hypothermia while maintaining a core temperature of 35-36°C (2).

2.1.2. After resuscitation

- **Mild EAI**: neonates can be transferred to the mother. These newborns should also be monitored frequently over the first 48 to 72 hours for any clinical abnormalities.
- **Moderate or severe AIS**: transfer to intensive care unit and neonatal resuscitation.

2.2. During hospitalization

Initial management of asphyxiated neonates after admission to the neonatal intensive care unit (NICU) is essential to prevent or reduce ongoing brain damage in asphyxiated neonates.

Temperature control, respiratory and cardiac support, treatment of seizures, maintenance of normal blood glucose, hematocrit and electrolytes, correction of blood gases and alterations in acid-base status, are all essential in the management of this category of neonates (6).

- **Temperature maintenance**
  - Conditioning on the heating table.
  - Maintain a normal temperature, avoid hyperthermia and especially hypothermia, which imposes additional stress by increasing metabolic requirements in the face of hypoxia-

ischemia. This can lead to acidosis, myocardial depression, hypotension, bleeding tendency and pulmonary hemorrhage (7).

- **Monitoring vital signs**

  Immediate clinical assessment of respiratory rate, heart rate, blood pressure, skin recolouration time (CRT), temperature and oxygen saturation, with diuresis monitoring.

- **Basic ration**

  Current recommendations aim to limit fluid intake. Restricting fluid intake can limit cerebral edema, which may play an important role in the pathogenesis of brain damage after perinatal asphyxia (8).

- **Respiratory management**

  Respiratory assistance is often required for newborns with EAI, due to the respiratory distress often associated with meconium aspiration syndrome and/or persistent pulmonary hypertension. It is important to ensure adequate ventilation, as variations in PCO2 can affect cerebral blood flow.

- **Blood tests**

  - Blood glucose: to detect hypoglycemia or hyperglycemia
  - CBC: look for thrombocytopenia, anemia or polycythemia
  - Blood gases: maintain blood gases and acid-base status within physiological norms: PaO2 between 80-100 mm

Hg; PaCO2 between 35-40 mm Hg and pH between 7.35-7.45.

- **Vascular filling**

  - If skin recoloration time (SRT) > 3 seconds or metabolic acidosis is present, volume expansion with 10 ml/kg saline over 5-10 min should be initiated.

  - Maintain mean arterial blood pressure (BP) above 35 mm Hg.Dopamine or dobutamine can be used to maintain adequate cardiac output if required.

- **Monitoring**

Vital parameter monitoring should be continued (9):

- Diuresis quantification
- Blood gas monitoring
- Blood glucose (2, 6, 12, 24, 48 and 72 hours)
- FNS, once a day for the first few days
- Serum sodium, potassium and calcium (once a day)
- Renal function: serum creatinine, creatinine clearance and urea
- Determination of cardiac and liver enzymes.
- Assessment of neurological status: tone, seizures, autonomic disturbances and archaic reflexes every 4-6 hours. At the end of this examination, EAI is classified as: mild, moderate and severe, using the Sarnat and Sarnat classification.

- **Management of convulsions**

Seizures can be subtle in character, so careful observation is needed to document them.

Treatment of neonatal seizures aims to prevent clinical deterioration, worsening brain damage and long-term neurodevelopmental problems, and to reduce the risk of future epilepsy (10).

The anticonvulsant of choice for seizure control is phenobarbital.

The initial dose is 20 mg/kg, given slowly intravenously over 20 minutes. If there is no response, two additional doses of 10 mg/kg each may be administered every 15 minutes. The phenobarbital infusion rate should not exceed 1 mg/kg/min, and it is preferable to use an electric syringe to administer the drug. For uncontrolled convulsions, add phenytoin sodium at a dose of 20 mg/kg intravenously, slowly over 20 minutes (11,12).

Recently, other anticonvulsants have been proposed. Topiramate has emerged as a potential anticonvulsant drug for neonates.

Levetiracetam is also a promising anticonvulsant drug that reduces excitotoxicity and does not induce neuronal apoptosis; but researchers have yet to evaluate its efficacy in large-scale clinical trials (13).

- The continuation of anticonvulsant treatment in the neonatal period is not recommended in practice, except for frequent clinical seizures (14).

2.3. Therapeutic hypothermia (HT)

Widespread adoption of this technique has been endorsed and incorporated by the International Liaison Committee on Resuscitation (ILCOR) and the American Academy of Pediatrics (AAP) since 2010 (14).

Currently, induced hypothermia is the only therapy considered beneficial. Various studies have shown that neonates with neonatal encephalopathy were treated with induced hypothermia to reduce mortality and neurological morbidity (15).

➢ **Neuroprotective effects**

HT has several beneficial effects: it reduces cerebral metabolism, prevents seizures, stabilizes the blood-brain barrier, inhibits glutamate and NO release, selectively reduces apoptosis and suppresses microglia activation (15).

➢ **Procedure**

Hypothermia is generally applied to a selected category of neonates meeting specific inclusion criteria. It should be started as soon as possible after birth in patients meeting the inclusion criteria.

➢ **Indications** (9)

To be effective, it should be started as soon as possible (between H2 and H6). If hypothermia is envisaged, contact the hypothermist as soon as possible.

neonatal intensive care unit to organize transport as quickly as possible.

a. **Target population**

- Gestational age ≥ 36 SA
- Birth weight ≥ 1800 g

b. **Exclusion criteria**

- Severe chromosomal or congenital anomalies
- Neurological trauma (severe intra- or extra-cerebral haemorrhage, spinal cord injury).
- Very severe hypoxoischemic encephalopathy for which palliative management is being considered

c. **Inclusion criteria**

Evaluation is based on 3 successive criteria: anamnestic (criteria A), clinical (criteria B) and electrophysiological (criteria C).

The combination of each of these criteria indicates that the patient should be placed in controlled hypothermia in a referral department.

A-Clinical and biological anamnestic criteria

Newborn ≥ 36 SA and weight ≥ 1800g born in the context of perinatal asphyxia with at least one of the following criteria:

1. Apgar ≤ 5 at M10

2. Respiratory resuscitation (tracheal intubation or mask ventilation) where

Cardiopulmonary still required at M10

3. Acidosis at cord or first hour of life (arterial, venous or capillary)

Defined by pH <7 and/or base deficit ≤ - 16 mmol/l and/or lactate levels ≥ 11 mmol/l

- In the absence of blood gas or in the event of a pH between 7.01 and 7.15, the child must have a history of perinatal asphyxia and meet criteria 1 or 2.
- If child meets A criteria, perform neurological assessment using B criteria

B- Clinical criteria

Moderate to severe encephalopathy **(Sarnat and Sarnat classification)** defined by a :

Lethargy (reduced response to stimuli) or coma (absent response to stimuli) and one or more of the following signs:

1. Hypotonia overall or limited to the upper part of the body
2. Abnormal reflexes: Moro (weak or absent) or oculomotor or pupillary abnormalities (constricted or dilated pupils not reactive)
3. Little or no suction
4. Clinical seizures

If the child meets criteria A and B, perform an electrophysiological evaluation with EEG and/or aEEG.

C. Criteria C

A 30-minute EEG or aEEG recording is required to continue hypothermia with background trace abnormalities plus at least one pejorative criterion:

- **EEG:**

- Paroxysmal trace without physiological figure

- Poor trace enriched with a few theta waves
- Track inactive
- Continuous critical activity

aEEG :

- Discontinuous trace - moderately abnormal - lower limit < 5μV and upper limit > 10 μV
- Discontinuous trace - severely abnormal - lower limit < 5μV and upper limit < 10μV
- Paroxysmal trace (burst suppression)
- Continuous critical activity

If criteria A+B+C are present, the child is treated with controlled hypothermia (rectal or esophageal temperature maintained at 33.5°C ± 0.5°C) for at least 72 hours after its initiation. Hypothermia can be discontinued if the EEG or aEEG are normal within the first 6 hours of life. In this case, slow rewarming over 6 hours is recommended.

Very gradual warming at H72 from onset of hypothermia:

- Risks of hypotension and convulsions if reheating is too rapid.
- Aim for +0.50°c/h maximum, i.e. at least 6 h
- Make stops in case of too rapid heating
- Beware of hyperthermia at the end of reheating and in the days that follow.
- The aim is to achieve a stable skin temperature of between 36 and 36.50°C.

There are two methods of active hypothermia treatment: selective head-cooling hypothermia and total body hypothermia.
The first modality involves external cooling of the head, while the second uses a small mattress filled with a cooling liquid that envelops the newborn's body.

In its current approach, therapeutic hypothermia aims to cool the newborn's body temperature to 33.5°C for 72 hours within 6 hours of birth, followed by gradual rewarming at a rate of 0.3°C to 0.5°C per hour (16).

- **Undesirable effects**

The most frequently observed are: pneumonia, thrombocytopenia, cardiac arrhythmia with prolongation of PR and QT intervals and sinus bradycardia, severe arterial hypotension.
(< 50mmHg), ionic disorders, pancreatitis and severe haemostasis disorders.

Controlled hypothermia above 33°C is recommended to avoid the deleterious side effects associated with lower temperatures (15).

A recent Cochrane review of 11 randomized controlled trials found that therapeutic hypothermia is beneficial in term newborns with EAI. Cooling was found to reduce mortality without increasing major disability in survivors (4).

2.4. Neuroprotective pharmacological agents

Although the pathophysiological features of EAI are complex, the multiple steps leading to cell damage offer numerous possibilities for therapeutic intervention. Various pharmacological pathways are currently being investigated. These include erythropoietin, melatonin, xenon, deferoxamine, topiramate and magnesium and stem cell therapy. Combining induced hypothermia with one of these drugs could improve the results obtained to date. Some of these molecules are promising, but further clinical studies are needed to determine the place of these potential neuroprotective agents in the drug arsenal for the treatment of neonatal hypoxic-ischemic encephalopathy (17).

References :

1. Executive summary: Neonatal encephalopathy and neurologic outcome, second edition.

   Report of the American College of Obstetricians and Gynecologists' Task Force on Neonatal Encephalopathy. Obstet Gynecol. 2014 Apr;123(4):896-901

2. Levy G, Bednarek N, Gabriel R. E. EM-Consulte. Per partum fetal asphyxia and conditions

   non-reassuring.

3. Rainaldi MA, Perlman JM. Pathophysiology of Birth Asphyxia. Clin Perinatol 1 Sept.

   2016 ;43(3):409-22.

4. Antonucci R, Porcella A, Pilloni MD. Perinatal asphyxia in the term newborn. J Pediatr Neonatal Individ Med . oct 2014;3(2):e030269

5. Wyckoff MH, Wyllie J, Aziz K, de Almeida MF, Fabres J, Fawke J, et al. Neonatal Life Support: 2020 International Consensus on Cardiopulmonary Resuscitation and Emergency Cardiovascular Care Science With Treatment Recommendations. Circulation. 20 Oct 2020;142(16_suppl_1):S185-221.

6. Wachtel EV, Hendricks-Muñoz KD. Current management of the infant who presents with neonatal encephalopathy. Curr Probl Pediatr Adolesc Health Care. 2011;41(5):132-53.

7. Antonucci R, Porcella A, Pilloni MD. Perinatal asphyxia in the term newborn. J Pediatr Neonatal Individ Med . oct 2014;3(2):e030269

8. Agarwal R, Jain A, Deorari AK, Paul VK. Post-resuscitation management of asphyxiated neonates. Indian J Pediatr. Feb 2008;75(2):175-80.

9. Meau-Petit V, Tasseau A, Lebail F, Ayachi A, Layouni I, Patkai J, et al. Controlled hypothermia of the term newborn after perinatal asphyxia. Arch Pediatrics March 2010;17(3):282-9.

10. Shetty J. Neonatal seizures in hypoxic-ischaemic encephalopathy - risks and benefits of anticonvulsant therapy. Dev Med Child Neurol . Apr 2015 ;57:40-3.

11. Glass HC, Ferriero DM. Treatment of hypoxic-ischemic

encephalopathy in newborns. Curr Treat Options Neurol . nov 2007];9(6):414-23.

12. Yozawitz E, Stacey A, Pressler RM. Pharmacotherapy for Seizures in Neonates with Hypoxic Ischemic Encephalopathy. Pediatr Drugs . dec 2017 ;19(6):553-67.

13. Douglas-Escobar M, Weiss MD. Hypoxic-Ischemic Encephalopathy: A Review for the Clinician. JAMA Pediatr . Apr 1, 2015 ;169(4):397.

14. De Caen AR, Kleinman ME, Chameides L, Atkins DL, Berg RA, Berg MD, et al. Part

10: Paediatric basic and advanced life support. Resuscitation [Internet]. oct 2010 ;81(1):e213-59.

15. Barrea C, Seghaye MC, Battisti O. Induced hypothermia in anoxoischemic encephalopathy of the newborn. 19(Percentile|Vol 19|N°1|2014):10-6.

16. Lutz IC, Allegaert K, de Hoon JN, Marynissen H. Pharmacokinetics during therapeutic hypothermia for neonatal hypoxic ischaemic encephalopathy: a literature review. BMJ Paediatr Open . June 2020 4(1):e000685.

17. Yildiz EP, Ekici B, Tatli B. Neonatal hypoxic ischemic

encephalopathy: an update on disease pathogenesis and treatment.

Expert Rev Neurother. May 2017;17(5):449-59.

Chapter 5

1. Evolution

1.1. In the short term

1.1.1. Risk of death

Neonatal asphyxia is a major cause of neonatal mortality. Death is directly correlated with the intensity and duration of asphyxia: in utero or in the delivery room, or after failed resuscitation (major hemodynamic failure), the reported mortality rate is around 20% in neonates asphyxiated at term (1) .

More than a third of live neonates admitted to intensive care with post-asphyxia encephalopathy are fatal (2).

A recent study published in Lancet showed the importance of the five-minute Apgar score in neonatal mortality, and demonstrated the role of the Apgar score in predicting neonatal mortality. A low 5-minute Apgar score was strongly associated with the risk of neonatal and infant death (3).

1.1.2. Multi-organ failure

In addition to brain damage, asphyxia can affect all organs, causing respiratory, renal, digestive, cardiac, hematological and metabolic failure, as well as skin lesions (bedsores and hypodermatitis).

The severity of hypoxic-ischemic encephalopathy has been shown to correlate strongly with multi-organ dysfunction in the first three days of life (4).

However, it has been found that there is no association between the presence of organ dysfunction and the long-term outcome of these newborns (5).

1.1.2.1. Kidney damage

Renal damage in perinatal asphyxia is the leading cause of multi-system damage. It follows severe renal hypo-perfusion, which if prolonged can lead to focal or diffuse alteration of the renal micro-vascularization, resulting in more or less extensive cortical necrosis (6).

There is no consensus on the definition of acute renal failure in newborns, making it difficult to estimate its incidence.

Oliguria is another clinical sign associated with AKI. However, in neonates, renal failure can occur in the absence of oliguria in over 50% of cases. Renal impairment in APN is mainly diuresis-preserved. Other clinical abnormalities of renal failure are rare in APN: hematuria, proteinuria and edema (6).

Studies have shown that ARF following birth asphyxia is positively correlated with the risk of morbidity and mortality in asphyxiated newborns (7) .

1.1.2.2. Liver damage

Birth asphyxia in neonates can cause hypoxic liver injury, resulting in the release of intracellular enzymes and a significant increase in their levels.

There is usually an early, abrupt and transient (within 24 to 72 hours) increase in various liver enzymes, namely aspartate aminotransaminase (ASAT), alanine amino-transaminase (ALAT), alkaline phosphatase (PAL) and lactate dehydrogenase (LDH). In general, these elevations normalize within 10 days of birth (8).

1.1.2.3. Heart disease

APN acts primarily on nervous tissue, but also on the heart, through

hypoxia and the resulting ischemia-reperfusion lesions. Myocardial development at birth is still incomplete and cannot respond adequately to this aggression. Some studies report that 78% of all babies with severe PA have suffered cardiac complications (9) .
Cardiac damage includes ventricular dysfunction, arrhythmia, sinus bradycardia and hypotension. Functional and conduction abnormalities can be detected by echocardiography and electrocardiogram, while heart muscle lesions are reflected by increased cardiac enzymes (troponins).

Despite the observation of these functional problems, the immediate and long-term structural consequences of birth in the context of asphyxia on the heart are not well understood (10).

1.1.2.4. Lung disease

Pulmonary impairment is defined by the need for > 40% oxygen ventilation support for at least the first 4 hours after birth (6).
The specific mechanisms underlying respiratory failure in asphyxiated neonates are manifold: fetal hypoxemia, ischemia, meconium aspiration, left ventricular dysfunction and coagulation defects.

On the other hand, perinatal asphyxia alters the complex physiological adaptation, hindering the fall in pulmonary resistances, which can lead to pulmonary hypertension (11) .

1.1.2.5. Digestive disease

Hypoxia is responsible for mucosal damage to the intestinal wall. Among the many digestive complications of asphyxia are ulcerative colitis, acute stomach necrosis and/or intestinal perforation.

The extent of lesions influences nutritional management. It is recommended to wait 3 days for mucosal lesions to heal and 7 days for more extensive lesions before attempting enteral feeding (12) .

1.1.2.6. Hematological disorders

The hematological system may also be affected. Asphyxia can alter the biophysical properties of blood, leading to changes in the properties, structure and functions of red blood cells and platelets. This also manifests itself as disseminated intravascular coagulation, with the need to administer labile blood products to prevent pulmonary or intracranial haemorrhage. In the event of ischemic bone marrow injury, the first sign will be thrombocytopenia around 5 to 7 days of age, as platelets have the shortest half-life of all marrow products (12,13).

1.1.2.7. Metabolic abnormalities

Hypoglycemia, hypocalcemia and inappropriate secretion of antidiuretic hormone leading to hyponatremia are the most common metabolic disorders in APN. These abnormalities must be treated to avoid aggravating the attacks (14) .

1.2. Long-term development

The neurological sequelae of perinatal asphyxia may give rise to several clinical pictures, associated or not, generally well correlated with the topography of the lesions.

IMOC, now called cerebral palsy (CP), results in motor disorders affecting movement and posture and/or impairment of certain cognitive functions.

Motor disorders, usually diagnosed within the first 18 months, can be :

- Limb paralysis, most often associated with spasticity of the affected muscles: Spastic CP.
- Abnormal movements: dyskinetic CP.
- Balance disorders: ataxic PC.

These different motor disorders may be associated, in which case we speak of mixed CP. Children with cerebral palsy are not a homogeneous population: some may suffer only a slight limp, while others will be severely handicapped and dependent on a third party for all acts of daily living.

Cognitive disorders are either intellectual deficiencies of varying intensity, as assessed by intelligence quotients, or neuropsychological disorders affecting specific areas of learning: dysphasia (language disorders), dyspraxia (gesture planning disorders), memory disorders, attention disorders, executive function disorders (ability to plan a task), which can lead to dyslexia, dyscalculia, dysgraphia and dysorthographia. Invisible in early childhood, these elective cognitive disorders are revealed as the child develops, in line with age-related expectations. They can be revealed by the more or less serious difficulties at school they generate in intelligent, motivated children. It is therefore important to diagnose them early and accurately (between the ages of 4 and 7). A neuropsychological assessment (15) is used to identify and analyze them.

Autism spectrum disorders, behavioral problems, hyperreactivity and psychotic symptoms, notably schizophrenia, have also been reported (16).

Clinically, damage to the basal ganglia and internal capsule in children born at term results in spastic quadriplegia with extension to oral and facial motor skills, and dystonic and dyskinetic disorders.

When there is cortico-subcortical damage, the IMOC picture is completed by cognitive impairment and mental retardation in 75% of cases, associated with microcephaly. Epilepsy is common in association with cortical damage. Sensory disorders are not uncommon, including blindness and deafness (17).

References

1. Antonucci R, Porcella A, Pilloni MD. Perinatal asphyxia in the term newborn. J Pediatr

   Neonatal Individ Med. oct 2014;3(2):e030269.

2. Pierrat V. Prevalence, causes, and outcome at 2 years of age of newborn encephalopathy: population based study. Arch Dis Child - Fetal Neonatal Ed . May 1, 2005 ;90(3):F257-f261.

3. Iliodromiti S, Mackay DF, Smith GCS, Pell JP, Nelson SM. Apgar score and the risk of cause-specific infant mortality: a population-based cohort study. The Lancet. nov 2014;384(9956):1749-55.

4. Alsina M, Martín-Ancel A, Alarcon-Allen A, Arca G, Gayá F, García-Alix A. Pediatr Crit Care Med [Internet]. march 2017 ;18(3):234-40.

5. Shah P. Multiorgan dysfunction in infants with post-asphyxial hypoxic-ischaemic encephalopathy. Arch Dis Child - Fetal Neonatal Ed [Internet]. March 1, 2004 ;89(2):152F - 155.

6. Durkan AM, Alexander RT. Acute Kidney Injury Post Neonatal Asphyxia. J Pediatr Feb 2011;158(2):e29-33.

7. La Rosa DA, Ellery SJ, Walker DW, Dickinson H. Understanding the Full Spectrum of Organ Injury Following Intrapartum Asphyxia. Front Pediatr. 17 Feb 2017;5.

8. Sharma D, Choudhary M, Lamba M, Shastri S. Correlation of Apgar Score with Asphyxial Hepatic Injury and Mortality in Newborns: A Prospective Observational Study From India. Clin Med Insights Pediatr. 2016;10:27-34.

9. Popescu MR, Panaitescu AM, Pavel B, Zagrean L, Peltecu G, Zagrean AM. Getting an Early Start in Understanding Perinatal Asphyxia Impact on the Cardiovascular System. Front Pediatr. 2020;8:68.

10. Polglase GR, Ong T, Hillman NH. Cardiovascular alterations and multi organ dysfunction after birth asphyxia. Clin Perinatol [Internet]. sept 2016;43(3):469-83.

11. Lapointe A, Barrington KJ. Pulmonary Hypertension and the Asphyxiated Newborn. J Pediatr . Feb 2011;158(2):e19-24.

12. Leuthner SR, Das U ("Shonu") G. Low Apgar scores and the definition of birth asphyxia. Pediatr Clin North Am . June 2004;51(3):737-45.

13. Brucknerová I, Ujházy E. Asphyxia in newborn - risk, prevention and identification of a hypoxic event. 2014;10.18

14. Thakur J, Bhatta NK, Singh RR, Poudel P, Lamsal M, Shakya A. Prevalence of electrolyte disturbances in perinatal asphyxia: a prospective study. Ital J Pediatr 21 May 2018 ;44

15. Bax M, Goldstein M, Rosenbaum P, Leviton A, Paneth N, Dan B, et al. Proposed definition and classification of cerebral palsy, April 2005. Dev Med Child Neurol . August 2005 ;47(8):571-6.

16. Perez A, Ritter S, Brotschi B, Werner H, Caflisch J, Martin E, et al. Long-Term Neurodevelopmental Outcome with Hypoxic-Ischemic Encephalopathy. J Pediatr . August 2013;163(2):454-459.e1.

18. Boog G. Perinatal asphyxia and cerebral palsy (I- The diagnosis). Gynécologie Obstétrique Fertil . avr 2010 ;38(4):261-77

Conclusion

Our journey through the twists and turns of perinatal asphyxia has come to an end, leaving us with a profound reflection on the issues surrounding this complex problem. Like a beacon in the night, this book has shed light on the causes, mechanisms, consequences and diagnostic methods of this condition, which unfortunately affects many newborns.

Beyond pure knowledge, the main aim of this book was to offer a perspective of hope and action. Indeed, while perinatal asphyxia can have serious consequences, it is important to emphasize that medical advances now make it possible to prevent, diagnose and manage it more effectively.

Prevention remains the fundamental pillar in the fight against perinatal asphyxia. Rigorous prenatal monitoring, adequate information for pregnant women and rapid management of obstetric complications are key to reducing the incidence of this condition.

Early and accurate diagnosis of perinatal asphyxia is also crucial to optimize the chances of survival and development of the newborn. Various assessment methods, such as fetal monitoring, blood gas analysis and medical imaging, enable healthcare professionals to rapidly identify at-risk cases and implement appropriate interventions.

The management of perinatal asphyxia requires a multidisciplinary approach involving paediatricians, neonatologists, anaesthetists and other specialists. Care of the newborn must be individualized and adapted to the severity of his or her condition, taking into account the potential risks and expected benefits of each intervention.

Support for families facing perinatal asphyxia is also an essential aspect of care. Parents must be offered appropriate psychological and emotional support, taking into account their specific experiences and needs.

In conclusion, perinatal asphyxia remains a major public health challenge, but advances in research and medical practice offer encouraging prospects for the future. By stepping up prevention efforts, improving diagnostic methods and optimizing care, we can considerably reduce the impact of this condition and offer the most fragile newborns the chance of a healthy life.

While not claiming to have all the answers, this book is a modest contribution to the fight against perinatal asphyxia. By sharing knowledge and raising awareness, we can all work towards a world where every birth is synonymous with hope and joy.

May this intellectual journey inspire and motivate you to commit yourself to this noble cause, such is the ambition of this book. Together, let's build a better future for newborns around the world.

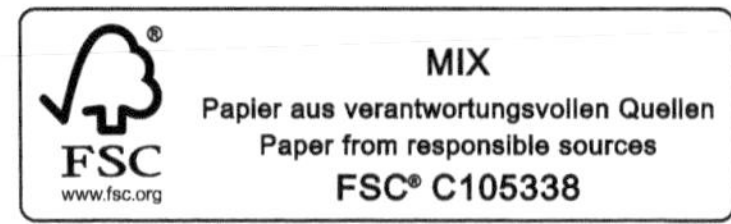

Printed by Books on Demand GmbH, Norderstedt / Germany